'To ensure that cardiac patients receive the best possible care during the worst possible times' - Adrian Levine & Joel Dunning

We are greatly indebted to the many hours of work put into the
creation of this course and this handbook by many clinicians including :
Madhav Menon, Rob Sinclair, Lea Callan, Jennine Stevenson, Karen Nixey, Bruce Atkins,
Matthew Bates, Amy Rogers, Christian Karcher, Savio Law, Andrew MacDonald, Neil Swanson,
Amelia Muir, David Lizotte, Adrian Levine, Joel Dunning

Index

Introduction

Can you think of a case in the catheter lab that went wrong ? Perhaps they arrested. Perhaps there was a tamponade or maybe they didn't even arrest but it was a tremendously stressful event for you and all the staff involved. Well you are not alone. We all have cases like this. Thankfully it is rare, but just because it is a rare event, we often make the mistake of going back to the way we normally work, dealing with large numbers of increasingly elderly and unwell patients, and that last traumatic and stressful case becomes a distant memory…. until the next time !

We have formed a group of dedicated clinicians who realise how different it is working in a modern catheter lab today. And like all fast changing environments, we face new and more difficult challenges while our hospitals become less accepting of complications. Together we feel that standard Adult Cardiac Life Support protocols are not fit for purpose in the catheter lab and we need our own way of dealing with the many very specific complications we face. We need to train and practice together as a team to make sure that these complications are dealt with quickly and efficiently according to protocols that we have agreed together in advance.

That is the basis for the REACT course. There are no new emergencies and people all over the world face these challenges every day, so we need to learn from each other and set out how to deal with a coronary vessel dissection, a tamponade after left atrial ablation, a left main stem occlusion in a TAVI case, and even the more common oversedation, pneumothorax, allergic reactions and many other less dramatic complications that if dealt with quickly and efficiently can lead to a quick recovery.

We also seek to use our worldwide network of clinicians to quickly learn from each other to make sure that our protocols are the best they can be and also to create not only in-person training but a range of online learning opportunities and forums to share our experiences.

We are delighted that you are joining this network and thank you for your interest in REACT. We already have so many real world examples of patients surviving their arrests due to this teamwork and practice that you are now embarking on. I hope you go on to encourage others to learn the protocols and practice too, and remember that we are a worldwide community so keep in touch with us and share your experiences with us so we can learn from you too.

Joel Dunning
Consultant at the James Cook University Hospital, Middlesbrough, UK
On behalf of all those involved in the REACT Course

Resuscitation and Acute Catheter Lab Emergencies

Rationale for a course

When I was a medical student in the John Radcliffe hospital in Oxford in 1994 the Cath lab was a very different place to the one it is today. We would go and watch long lines of 50 year old men undergoing femoral access diagnostic angiograms, and, just to show us that there was variety in a cardiologists life, we were shown some pacemaker insertions too ! It is quite stunning to think that two decades later we are performing regular multivessel PCI including in complex lesions and occluded vessels, we now perform large numbers of PCIs acutely, and in the middle of the night, in very unwell patients, we have biventricular ICDs , wireless pacing systems, complex ablation procedures, watchman devices to reduce the risk of stroke, and of course the explosion of valve interventions on the aortic, mitral and pulmonary valves which are rapidly becoming routine.

But with every new development comes new risks and complications, and each of these complications needs a highly skilled team to be able to work together to address the issues.

It was our experience talking to clinicians of all types in the catheter labs that led us to believe that the cardiologist was often the key to remedying the complication, but their actions would require their full and undivided attention to make sure they succeed. Whether this is placement of a covered stent in a dissection, or a pericardial drain for tamponade, or addressing a compromised left main stem in a TAVI, they need to remain scrubbed by the side of the patient while a team around them took care of the resuscitation of the patient. And if we trained a team around them to work efficiently and reliably to resolve the situation, according to a well-tested set of emergency protocols, then this would significantly reduce the risks of mistakes and allow a calm environment to work in. In addition we felt that staff working in the catheter labs are best placed to address most of the complications that we see. Often hospital resuscitation teams, if called into this alien environment, are well out of their depth, do not feel able to take over from a consultant cardiologist, are not aware about the need to wear lead aprons and would have no knowledge about specialist interventions needed to resolve the situation. Therefore we need to think carefully about who we call to the catheter labs in emergencies and how we utilise them safely and make sure they feel confident and informed enough to support us.

The Principles of React

We have a series of principles that guide the rationale for our protocols.

The first one is :

An Emergency is not the time to test your memory

I think that historically, life support courses have been conducted worldwide where at the end of the day there is an individual clinician test which is pass or fail. This had involved memorising the whole guideline and demonstrating that you knew whether you gave the adrenaline at the end of the 3rd cycle or just before the 4th and a host of other facts and details. This has led to many staff members feeling that they are very bad at resuscitation or that resuscitation is difficult especially if they fail a course and have to retake it. We strongly feel that in an emergency it is necessary for us to have all the resources right to hand to look up the correct protocol and that as we are in a contained environment of the catheter lab and with modern technology such as apps on phones readily available, nobody should feel that they cannot just get the resources out and look up the agreed protocol, and we in fact actively mandate this in the course.

Our second principle is :

An emergency is not the time to discuss how to deal with one

We should be practising for all possible emergency scenarios together as a team in the simulation centre and that we should therefore all be aware of what will be done in that emergency once it arises in clinical practise. Clinicians have historically been far behind other specialties in simulation. Pilots have to log many hours per year in simulators in order to maintain their qualifications to fly. An athlete trains for about 90% of his career for only 10% of racing and military special forces train for 99% of their career for only 1% in live battle. Therefore we must regard this as part of our career not an optional extra.

We are letting our patients down by not making time in our clinical work for simulation. There is a whole host of novel ways we can do this and it does not require us to close a cath lab every week. We can use the online world and e-learning, we can discuss emergency situations in offices together or next to simulation manikins, and hopefully in the near future we can use virtual reality to simulate patients who become acutely unwell. But we do need to regularly come together to practise together as realistically as possible in the cath lab to put that groundwork together as a team.

Our third principle is :

Every emergency should have a standalone protocol

We must carefully consider every emergency situation and we must plan for it. Then if we have a full range of protocols then we can make them widely available. Anyone in the catheter lab can activate the protocol that is being faced and the protocols must be easily accessible to all members of the team. The advantage of not having to memorise the protocols is that we can then have a larger range of them and we can have them in as much detail as we wish. Practise and training can then concentrate on making sure that each protocol is fit for purpose and tailored to our own needs.

Our fourth principle is :

'Communication is key'.

We will discuss the REACT communication board later in this handbook, but a team briefing and a clear board in the catheter lab setting out a range of important clinical information will greatly assist in emergency situations. Also we must learn to communicate as a team throughout the procedure. There is a fixed hierarchy in all catheter labs but any member of the team might identify a critical error or a mistake, or may have a concern. We have to foster an open environment where the first year nursing student feels able to ask a question of the professor of cardiology and expect to be heard. We must also practice our emergency communication skills as this is not something we should assume just happens. Try to remember the last emergency situation that you were in. Quite often there may be one person in the room running the emergency and nobody else speaks, and many people are independently doing tasks that they think might help the situation without actively communicating them to the team leader. We need to make sure we have practiced active followership as well as leadership so that the leader if constantly being informed about what everyone around them is doing.

Our final principle is :

We need an advanced leadership structure in the catheter labs

This means that although the cardiologist remains in charge, and has ultimate responsibility for the care of the patient, we need a second leader in the room in an emergency to organise the team around them. The Cardiologist must be freed up to perform technically difficult tasks that only they can perform such as emergency PCI or pericardiocentesis. They also need to remain scrubbed by the patient's side, or they may need to concentrate on performing an echocardiogram. But this person cannot be distracted by needing to run the team around them to follow one of the known emergency protocols. A second team leader therefore should take charge of the resuscitation, ensuring that airway, breathing and circulation is optimised, that defibrillation is utilised and that specialist resources as called for as appropriate as specified in the protocols. This advanced leadership structure frees up the specialist cardiologist to perform tasks that only they can perform, while a well-trained team led by a second team leader resuscitates the patient, using the protocols that they have practiced.

The 6 Key Roles

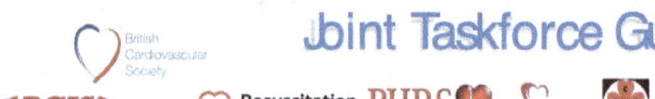
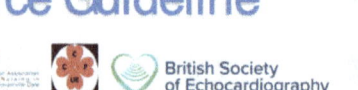
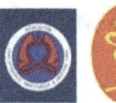
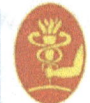
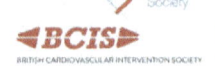
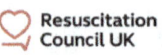
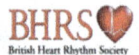

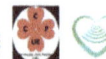
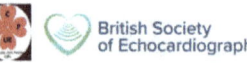

1. Emergency leader
2. Airway and breathing
3. Defibrillation and pacing
4. Manual CPR
5. Mechanical CPR, drugs and timing
6. Resource coordinator

Op: Operator
A : Assistant

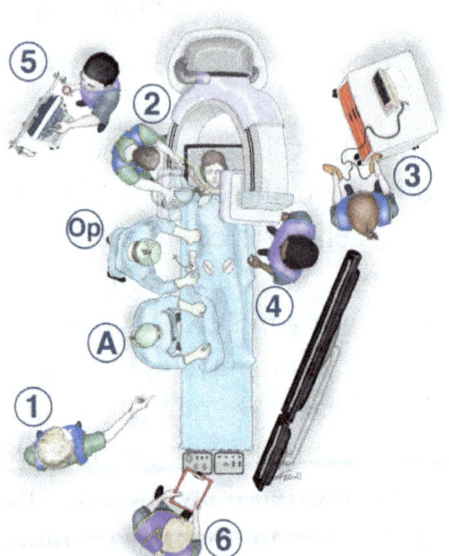

Introduction

In order to carry out all emergency protocols efficiently, whether they be an arrest situation or just an acute emergency it is vital for everyone to know their role. There may be a wide variety of numbers and skill mixes in the catheter labs depending on the size of the institution and also the time of day or night and therefore there will clearly also have to be some flexibility with these roles and also additional roles that might be allocated, but we have developed the 6 key roles to try to allow a structure for people to work towards. In addition we hope that the staff members will know in advance the role that they would be expected to take in an emergency, and that this should be documented on the communication board at the start of a shift.

The Operator

In fact while the cardiologist is the natural leader in the catheter lab, the main aim of our protocols is to free this person up of duties in the cardiac arrest or the emergency situation. The cardiologist should stay scrubbed at the side of the patient. They are often the person to see the emergency first, and thus must declare this early to the team. For example it is very important to tell your team what is happening i.e. 'I think we have a coronary vessel dissection', or 'I think this patient has a tamponade. It is often tempting as the clinician who may have caused the complication to try not to make too much of it, or communicate the problem late, but in fact for the safety of the patient this has to happen early.

The next task is just to make sure that an emergency leader is allocated. For example if the registrar is the emergency leader, then the cardiologist must state – 'we have a complication, can you take charge as the emergency leader'. Depending on local resources the cardiologist then may require the support of another team member to be scrubbed if they do not have a 3rd person scrubbed already. Team training makes this requirement very clear in each catheter lab. The cardiologist is best placed to perform the specialist interventions that may resolve the situation. Thus if there is a coronary vessel dissection, the cardiologist will be concentrating on the equipment and methods that he needs to use to get this emergency dealt with percutaneously. The Cardiologist will be thinking about which covered stent he needs and whether he needs a pericardial drain. It is important for his team to be dealing with the patient in terms of airway, breathing, defibrillation and circulation.

Role 1: The Emergency Leader

Our core principle is that of the advanced leadership structure, and thus having someone other than the cardiologist to organise the team to achieve the best outcome for the patient we feel is the key to a successful resuscitation model in the catheter labs. Importantly we do not mandate who this person should be in terms of qualifications and in fact we feel that everyone who works in a catheter lab should be trained to be able to carry out each of the 6 key roles. As we will discuss subsequently, this role would already have been allocated at the start of the shift on the communication board but if this has not happened then anyone in the room should feel that they should be able to perform this role and should clearly announce that they are taking the role so there is clarity from the team as to who the leader is.

The role is in fact quite simple in that for arrests the REACT arrest protocol is followed and the leader is encouraged to have it to hand on the flipchart, and in all the other acute emergencies, similarly, we encourage the use of flipcharts or folders containing the protocols. And therefore the emergency leader's main skill is to keep the team calm and focused and to make sure that everyone is doing their role efficiently, and to act as the central communication hub for the team. Thus in training, the emergency leader should go round each of his team in term, asking them what they have done so the team can be confident that each role is being carried out correctly. Thus the team leader should state 'John – how is the airway and breathing', to which it is hoped that the response will be 'I am getting good air entry at 100% oxygen. I have listened to the chest and I don't think there is a pneumothorax or haemothorax. I am happy'.

We would like the Emergency leader to be verbalising the next steps in the arrest or emergency protocols. Thus if we are in VF and are doing CPR, the team leader might say to the team, 'once we are at 2 minutes, I want John who is managing the airway to step back with the bag/valve/mask, I will ask Jane to charge the defibrillator to 200 joules while Ben continues massage, then I will ask Ben to stand back and we will deliver the shock. If it doesn't work we will all continue with the 2nd Cycle of CPR, is everyone happy with that ?

The Emergency leader will also allocate tasks to additional people to come to the room, outside of the 6 key roles and anyone entering the room should report to them. Thus if an anaesthetist comes into the room, the emergency leader can meet them, they can read the case notes off the communication board including important information that the anaesthetist will want to know. The team leader can also tell the anaesthetist whether lead aprons may be required if some fluoroscopy is expected. The REACT Course assumes that fluoroscopy may well be part of the emergency situation so we recommend that everyone places lead aprons on unless there is a particular reason not to. If further people come into the room then the emergency leader can either utilise them or actually telling someone they are not needed is very useful as that person will not then just be standing there watching, feeling that they should be doing more. We also have a resource commander role which we will describe who can also deal with the allocation of personnel and the briefing of key people, while they put on lead aprons.

Role 2: Airway and Breathing

If there is any acute emergency and especially in an arrest, the scrubbed personnel will be dealing with the circulation and role 1 is dealing with external cardiac massage, so the next most important role is that of airway and breathing. A person should go straight to the head of the patient to perform their tasks.

For a person not breathing they must immediately get a bag/valve/mask at 100% oxygen and place this on the patients face and attempt to ventilate the patient. If they are successful, then the chest will rise on both sides, and water vapour may be seen in the mask. If they are unsuccessful then an airway obstruction issue must be considered. Attempt airway manoeuvres – jaw thrust, chin lift, guedel airway and perhaps ask another person to help with squeezing the bag so you can use 2 hands to form a good seal around the patients nose and mouth may be required. We do not recommend intubation if you are not used to doing this. Most of the time simple airway manoeuvres and airway adjuncts will suffice. If the patient has a heavy beard then sleek or tape can be used to cover the beard around the mouth so a better seal is formed.

Once air entry is established in an arrest you must coordinate 30:2 with the person performing massage. Your role also requires you to feel the trachea to see if it is central or displaced and then ask everyone to stop massage once and bag forcefully while listening bilaterally to see if you can hear a difference in breath sounds.

It is mandatory to exclude a pneumothorax and haemothorax in every critically ill catheter lab patient and communicate that you have done this to the team leader. It can be quite difficult to do, but if you are getting air entry from bagging but it is more difficult than you would expect, if the trachea is not central and if you bag vigorously to try to hear breath sounds but cannot hear any on one side then that is your best chance of making the diagnosis of pneumothorax. We have one novel recommendation in the catheter lab and that is to take an AP fluoroscopy image once for every arrested patient. The aim of this is not to see if we can identify a small pneumothorax, but to exclude a very large pneumothorax or tension pneumothorax that might be the cause of this arrest. The reason for recommending this is entirely because it is so difficult to listen for breath sounds and exclude a pneumothorax from clinical signs in an arrest situation.

We feel that a single fluoroscopy view just after the second cycle of CPR will be very quick and easy and relatively low in radiation and if it sees a large pneumothorax that caused the arrest this could be lifesaving. We feel that it could potentially also show an unexpectedly large pericardium too which might lead the team to be concerned about a tamponade and speed up the request for an echo. This step would not be necessary in arrests where the cause is clearly known like a vessel occlusion but for an unexpected arrest we feel that it is an important step.

If you suspect a pneumothorax but are not sure, i.e. a pacing procedure, and the sats dropped initially, and the patient complained of being short of breath before becoming in extremis, then it is probably safer to intervene and do a needle thoracocentesis followed by a drain, than not intervene as a drain in a person without a pneumothorax is safer than no drain in a patient with a tension pneumothorax!

We will address this further in the respiratory emergency protocol.

If you are in a prolonged emergency, then preparations will need to be made to intubate and ventilate the patient. If you are getting good air entry and good chest movement, you should not do this yourself unless you are an experienced anaesthetist, as it is much more difficult in an emergency situation and you might turn a stable situation into a 'can't intubate-can't ventilate' emergency. But in your role you can remind the emergency leader to get people to prepare the emergency airway trolley, the ventilator, and the drugs and equipment needed for intubation by the anaesthetist.

Role 3: Defibrillation and Pacing

We recommend that a single person is always allocated to this role and stays besides the defibrillator at all times, even if the rhythm is not VF or pulseless VT. The person fulfilling role 3 should place pads on the patient wherever it is most convenient. Often they will be draped and therefore access will be limited but this will have been practiced in simulation so this should not be an issue. Role 3 must announce that they are charging the defibrillator, then make sure everyone stands clear and removes all loose oxygen by facemask prior to administering defibrillation. If the patient is already intubated such as a complex ablation or TAVI then the breathing circuit does not need to be disconnected prior to defibrillation and it is actually more dangerous to do this.

We recommend 3 stacked shocks and this is supported in resuscitation guidelines in specialist areas, so once the first shock has been delivered, external cardiac massage should not be recommenced, but the rhythm assessed. As soon as it is clear that it has not succeeded then the defibrillator person must again announce that they are charging, and then shocking, and this should be done quickly a third time if return of spontaneous circulation is not achieved.

If the shock is successful then we would not recommend 2 minutes of massage while they are in sinus rhythm. This is in contrast to the ALS protocol which recommends a shock then 2 minutes of massage before a pulse check. The reason that we recommend this change is that our patients are likely to have been identified as having arrested immediately so their hearts will not be as distended as standard patients on a ward or out of hospital. Secondly many of our patient will have their arterial pressure being transduced and thus we are able to see what their blood pressure is. The ALS recommendation is for the benefit of patients with a delay to defibrillation whereby the heart becomes distended and therefore even in sinus rhythm they may not return their spontaneous circulation and 2 minute of massage can be effective in decompressing the heart. In contrast we can closely watch our blood pressure return and the heart will not be distended and therefore we are much more likely to achieve a good blood pressure immediately after successful defibrillation.

If the 3rd shock fails, massage must be recommenced. Then 2 minutes should be timed until the next time a shock is delivered. However the first 3 shocks are most likely to be effective and once we are down to the 4th shock the chance of success is diminished and thus we now revert to single shocks followed by massage for two minutes as recommended by the general algorithm. If 3 shocks or even more do not convert the VF or pulseless VT then the diagnosis is much more likely to be a structural heart issue causing the ischaemic VF rather than a simple arrhythmia, and thus tamponade or coronary vessel occlusion causing myocardial ischaemia should be carefully considered.

We should remember that most defibrillators when turned on activate a timer which is displayed clearly on the screen (Although most people don't realise this until it is pointed out !). Thus it may be that the person on defibrillation will also be the best person to time the CPR cycles. This is why it is on the defibrillator and thus communication with the team leader can establish early who is going to perform the timing role.

Role 3 is also important in the two other rhythm disturbances. In asystole or extreme bradycardia without a pulse then temporary pacing may rapidly resolve the situation in an arrest. We recommend that the pads are quickly placed on the patient, and it is also important to remember that defibrillators cannot pace and sense from the same pads and thus it is MANDATORY that ECG leads are placed on the patient and connected to the defibrillator prior to attempting to start pacing. We recommend that external cardiac massage is withheld until the pacing is attempted and in fact percussion pacing is tried rather than cardiac massage initially. When the pacing is activated on the defibrillator it usually defaults to the minimum amplitude, and therefore this will have to be turned up to the maximal possible amplitude to see if it will work. If it does not work at maximum amplitude then it is unlikely to work unless the pads are poorly placed and thus the attempt can cease. Of note the general ALS algorithm does not support the use of Atropine in an arrest and thus it is also not in our algorithm. If it is felt likely that the asystole could be resolved with pacing and the external pacing was unsuccessful then the final option would be a temporary wire to be placed in an arrest situation. With percussion pacing, external pacing and temporary wire placement we hope that in fact external cardiac massage would not be needed at all in the initial resuscitation of a patient with asystole.

The 3rd arrest rhythm is PEA. There is no role for the person allocated to defibrillation other than just to make sure that no mistake has been made by the team in thinking a rhythm with VF or asystole is in fact PEA from any pacing that is being given. We are aware of 3 cases when this occurred and although rare, if there is a temporary wire with pacing this can be paused to check, or if there is a permanent pacemaker then it the narrow nature of the 'QRS' seen regularly at around 60bpm should raise this suspicion. This is a busy role and this person has one more role to fulfil unless there are enough people for the team leader to allocate this to someone else:

Use varies quite widely around the world but many centres use automated compression devices successfully in established cardiac arrests. We recommend strongly the use of Mechanical CPR devices in all arrests in the catheter laboratory. The illustrations below demonstrate the LUCAS device, the 'Thumper' and the autopulse by ZOLL. Training and practice with the devices makes their use possible and allows the resuscitation to continue for longer periods of time more successfully especially if a team might consider the use of extracorporeal CPR, which may take some time to institute or need to perform PCI in an arrest. Of note multiple current guidelines including our own do recommend the use of automated CPR devices in the catheter lab and therefore we believe that they should be a standard piece of resuscitation equipment in catheter labs.

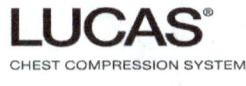

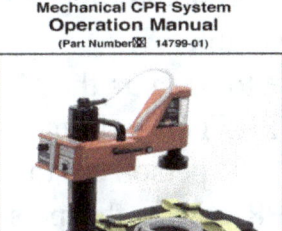

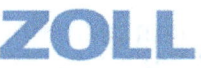

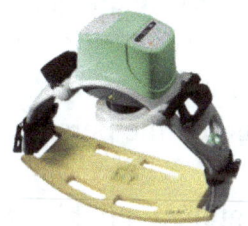

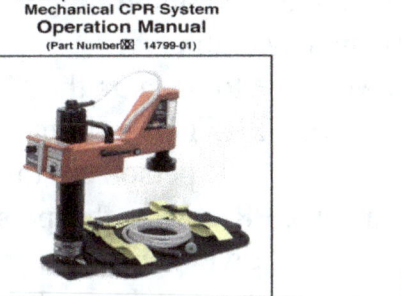

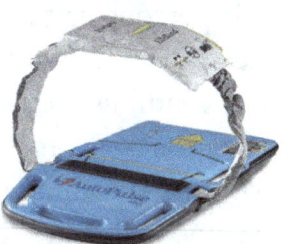

Role 4: Manual CPR

We need to allocate one person to perform CPR when required. If there are very limited numbers of people in the room at night then either the cardiologist or the scrub nurse could do this but it is an important role and having an allocated person is most preferable.

CPR is withheld if the arrest is VF or asystole until DC shocks have been administered or the external pacing has been turned on but if this has failed then CPR must be commenced. The person performing CPR will most likely need to be on the opposite side of the table to the cardiologist, and if the table is fairly high they may need a step to stand on. Hands should be linked together and elbow straight and CPR is performed on the midpoint of the sternum.

The general algorithm recommends a depth of 5-6cm and there are devices available to measure whether you are compressing adequately, but if your patient has an arterial line in place then in fact this can function as a direct measure of the quality of your CPR. If you have an arterial line then in preference to the depth recommendation you should compress the heart hard enough that you achieve a systolic pressure of 70mmHg. It is also important to note that if you have a well-functioning arterial line and you are compressing as hard as you can but you are unable to achieve a systolic pressure of 70mmHg this implies that there is a mechanical cause to the arrest such as a tamponade or a bleed, as this means that either the heart is compressed by tamponade and cannot fill with blood to eject as you compress, or that the heart is empty of blood due to blood loss. The Inability to perform CPR with a systolic of above 70mmHg is an emergency and requires you to immediately notify the team leader and cardiologist.

Role 4: Mechanical CPR drugs and timing

We feel that there is always a balance in protocols in terms of the detail that they should go to. Some smaller centres or primary PCI sites in the middle of the night will certainly not have 6 people in the catheter lab, but many busy catheter labs in the middle of the day will have large numbers of people immediately available. Therefore we considered protocols from 4 to 8 allocated members and we settled on 6 roles. The role of having a person in charge of mechanical CPR, drug administration, vascular access and timing we would regard as highly desirable assuming there is adequate personnel available.

Initially this persons first role would be to open up the Mechanical CPR device and get it ready to be placed after the first round of CPR. This is in fact a 3 person activity but the person on airway and breathing and the manual CPR person are the ideal 3 person team for this.

After application of the mechanical CPR device, this person would stand by the person allocated to airway and breathing and would give mediations as per protocol.

There are some key drugs that this person would need to have immediately available. Adrenaline (Epinephrine) in an arrest should be given at a dose of 1mg every 3-5 minutes. We mandate its administration after the 3rd cycle in the protocol. This will allow its administration at about 4-5 minutes into the arrest and therefore would be in line with all major guidelines. Also it is a convenient time to give it. In a VF arrest you would come to the end of the 3rd cycle of massage, you would charge the defibrillator up while massaging and give a shock and if this failed then the adrenaline should be given and CPR recommenced . Of note it should then be given every other cycle which is again in line with the general ALS algorithm.

We mandate its administration after the 3rd cycle in the protocol. This will allow its administration at about 4-5 minutes into the arrest and therefore would be in line with all major guidelines. Also it is a convenient time to give it. In a VF arrest you would come to the end of the 3rd cycle of massage, you would charge the defibrillator up while massaging and give a shock and if this failed then the adrenaline should be given and CPR recommenced . Of note it should then be given every other cycle which is again in line with the general ALS algorithm.

Many meta-analyses[1] and a recent very large study called PARAMEDIC-2[2] have all struggled to prove a significant benefit for adrenaline in arrests, with a number needed to treat of 112 in the PARAMEDIC-2 trial in order to see a benefit, (with worse neurological outcomes in those additional survivors), but nevertheless it is probably the most well-established drug in arrests and therefore a key part of the algorithm. Of note if the arrest is due to a resolvable mechanical issue such as a tamponade that needs draining, it may be best to withhold the adrenaline to avoid its proarrhythmic effects and indeed to cause HYPERtension once the tamponade is removed which may risk further bleeding from the vessel that caused the tamponade in the first place.

The second drug in VF arrest is Amiodarone. It has been shown to have a 10% increased change of defibrillation being successful in several RCTs and is recommended in all algorithms after the 3rd cycle. For the convenience of administration and to be as accurate as possible we have mandated it also after the 3rd cycle.

The 3rd drug to mention in cardiac arrests is Atropine. It was taken off the universal algorithm in 2015 due to lack of efficacy in the arrest situation and therefore it does not appear in our arrest algorithm either. It is important to remember that it is still an important medication in bradycardia when the patient has not arrested and it is recommended at a dose of 600mcg, repeated up to 3mg if the patient has a pulse. This issue has caused some confusion in the past.

Finally it is useful to mention that in cases of oversedation then naloxone at a dose of 400mcg repeated every 3minutes up to 10mg will immediately reverse the effects of morphine and fentanyl, and flumazenil at 200mcg iv repeated every 30 seconds up to 3mg will equally effect a rapid reversal of midazolam and other benzodiazepines.

In this role it is important to document the administration of all drugs and for patients with inadequate vascular access, perhaps such as a patient bleeding during a pacemaker insertion, then they may well be able to identify this problem and seek additional vascular access if they are adequately trained to do this.

As this person will have a role in documentation of the medications and the timing of administration it would seem a natural extension of this role to be the arrest timer if there is not an actual timer running on the defibrillator.

Role 5: Resource Coordinator

There are often many members of the team available to help in an emergency situation and on simulations and observations of real world emergencies it is clear that there has to be a great deal of organisation behind actual arrest or acute emergency. The Emergency Team leader needs to be by the patient and coordinating everything in the room but there have to be advanced lines of communication between the catheter lab, the CCU, the arrest team, the ICU, echocardiographers, and also other clinicians in the other catheter labs.

Therefore we feel this line of communication is sufficiently important to have a specific allocated role. In addition there is often a control room in the cath labs which has staff by the phones and in communication with the cath lab or a radiographer in the cath lab who can control the fluoroscopy when required but also make calls to teams in the hospital.

The role is straightforward as again the REACT Protocol is followed and on the flipcharts they specify actions, people and equipment needed for each emergency and thus this person can go smoothly down the list making sure all these resources are available.

We recommend that this person would be the ideal gatekeeper into the cath lab. If emergency personnel arrive, then the resource coordinator can hand them lead aprons (and remind them that they must be worn) and while they are being put on then they can brief the person as to the personnel arrive, then the resource coordinator can hand them lead aprons (and remind them that they must be worn) and while they are being put on then they can brief the person as to the case and what the nature of the emergency is. They may also be able to direct them to look at the communication board and to go and see the emergency leader rather than going into the room and immediately talking to the cardiologist.

Furthermore they may be an ideal person to hold the flipcharts of the emergency protocols. They may have time to look down these and to remind the Emergency leader of any important points listed in the agreed protocols.

The Arrest Protocol

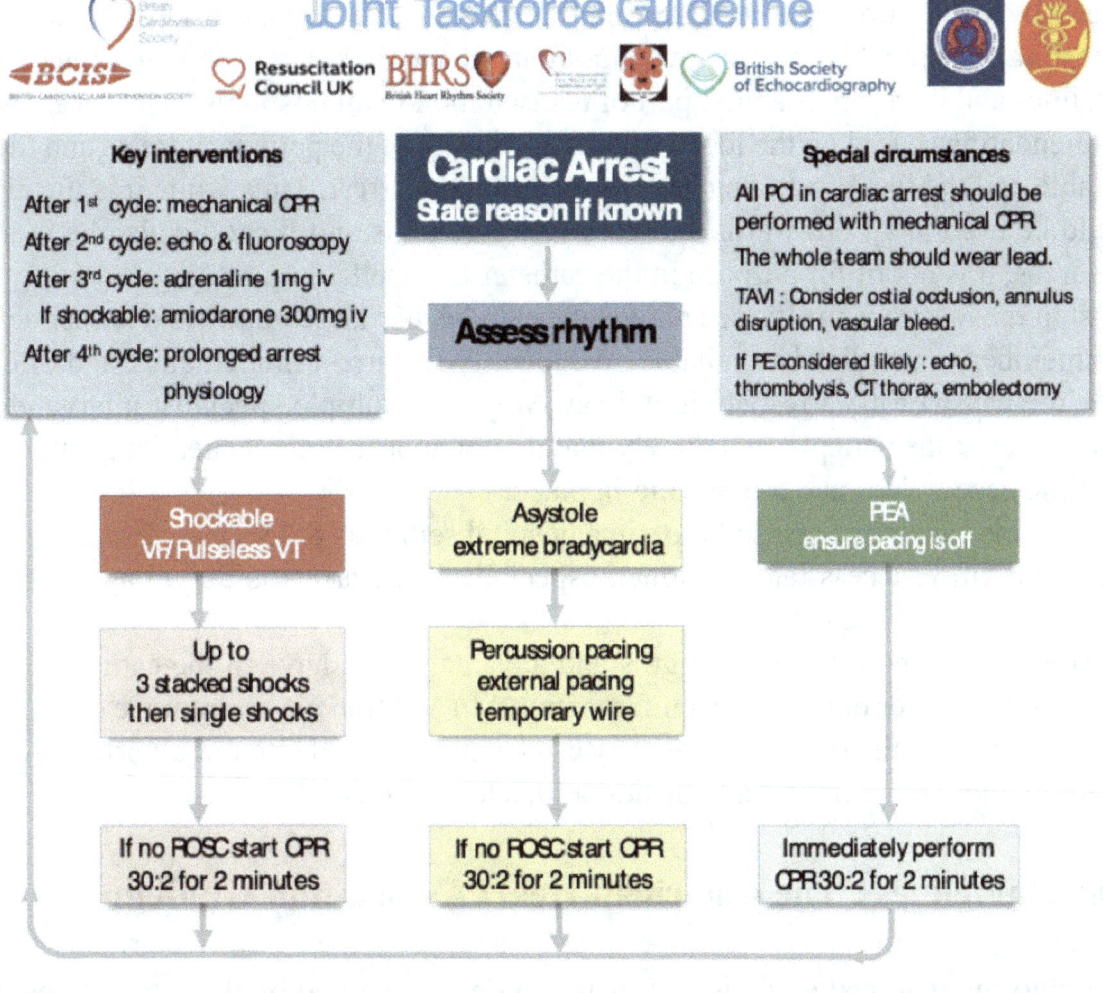

Joint Taskforce Guideline

Key interventions

After 1st cycle: mechanical CPR

After 2nd cycle: echo & fluoroscopy

After 3rd cycle: adrenaline 1mg iv

If shockable: amiodarone 300mg iv

After 4th cycle: prolonged arrest physiology

Cardiac Arrest
State reason if known

Assess rhythm

Special circumstances

All PCI in cardiac arrest should be performed with mechanical CPR

The whole team should wear lead.

TAVI : Consider ostial occlusion, annulus disruption, vascular bleed.

If PE considered likely : echo, thrombolysis, CT thorax, embolectomy

Shockable VF/ Pulseless VT	Asystole extreme bradycardia	PEA ensure pacing is off
Up to 3 stacked shocks then single shocks	Percussion pacing external pacing temporary wire	
If no ROSC start CPR 30:2 for 2 minutes	If no ROSC start CPR 30:2 for 2 minutes	Immediately perform CPR 30:2 for 2 minutes

Established arrest

CALL ARREST TEAM

Airway Breathing:
100% oxygen, protect airway.
Consider fluoroscopy for pneumothorax.
Obtain central venous access.
Take a blood gas

Circulation
Is there a haemothorax, retroperitoneal haematoma, pericardial collection, or aortic dissection?

Consider anaphylaxis
adrenaline 0.5mg IM, or 50mcg IV

Consider extracorporeal CPR

Prolonged arrest parameters

We recommend that teams consider recording the following parameters during prolonged cardiac arrest. Green, amber and red indicate potential impact of the physiological parameters achieved during cardiac arrest on ROSC and could be used to guide future research.

Systolic BP	60	70	80
Diastolic BP	25	30	40
ETCO$_2$ {kPa}	1.3	2.0	2.7
pH	7.0	7.1	7.2
Base Excess	-10	7.5	-5
SaO$_2$ %	70	80	90

Adjust CPR device, modify ventilation, consider inotropes, correct acidosis, optimize volume to achieve goals.

Return of spontaneous circulation

ABCDE approach
Keep SpO$_2$ 94-98%
Normalise PaCO$_2$
Consider inotropic support

Consider angiogram and Echo once ROSC established

Consider long term follow up of patients who arrest in the catheter lab to identify neurological and psychological sequelae

The differences between universal algorithms and the REACT Protocol

The Adult Advanced Life Support Algorithm that governs the management of arrests throughout our hospitals is probably the most well thought out and most intensively written of all medical guidelines and therefore is a vital part of resuscitation in all hospitals. But it is an evolution of recommendations based on the location of the majority of the patients it treats and the staff it has available and the likely pathology that has caused the arrest. Thus while it is the algorithm that should be used in all our wards and coronary care units and it should also be used in our recovery areas, it is not fit for purpose in the catheter lab itself.

In contrast to the locations mentioned above, the cath lab has large numbers of expert clinicians and staff members immediately available. We identify the arrest immediately and often we in fact know the cause of the arrest straight away. We have multiple specialist interventions that we can use to treat the patient immediately that do not appear in the general algorithm and we have multiple access lines and monitoring in place.

Finally while the success of resuscitation in a hospital setting is 8-15%, we should be planning on achieving a 50% success rate or higher, especially if the arrest is due to an interventional complication in an elective patient.

Our algorithm must optimise the strengths and advantages we have in the cath labs and must allow additional time for our specialist interventions. In addition we can remove or significantly modify factors such as the H's and T's as they can be incorporated into our algorithm which will save time and allow more important considerations to be included.

Current Guidelines : The American Heart Association Guidelines

With regard to International guidelines, Resuscitation is governed by the International Liaison Council on Resuscitation (ILCOR) which is a collaborative of 7 world resuscitation councils which was set up in 1992. Every 5 years the full range of all recommendations in resuscitation is reviewed and updated completely and a document of the 'best evidence' in resuscitation is created. The 7 resuscitation councils then take this evidence and generate their own guidelines adapted to the needs of their own healthcare systems.

Thus the American Heart Association and also the European Resuscitation council both have sections in their 2015 guidelines derived from the same evidence but they are relatively different in their text.

We have provided the text from both these guidelines in full due to their importance in relation to our protocols starting with the American guidelines. The American guidelines have chosen to mainly concentrate on a discussion with regard to automated CPR devices over manual compressions and also the use of extracorporeal CPR (ECPR) devices. No other structural changes to how we work in the cath labs are discussed.

Part 10.5: Cardiac Arrest During Percutaneous Coronary Intervention ALS 479
2015 American Heart Association Guidelines Update for Cardiopulmonary Resuscitation and
Emergency Cardiovascular Care
Eric J. Lavonas, Chair; Ian R. Drennan; Andrea Gabrielli; Alan C. Heffner; Christopher O.
Hoyte; Aaron M. Orkin; Kelly N. Sawyer; Michael W. Donnino.
Circulation. 2015;132[suppl 2]:S501–S518.

Cardiac arrest during PCI is rare, occurring in approximately 1.3% of catheterization procedures.[3,4] Although the risk of cardiac arrest during PCI is present in both elective and emergency procedures, the incidence is higher in emergency cases.[5] In general, patients who develop cardiac arrest during PCI have superior outcomes to patients in cardiac arrest that occurs in other settings, including in-hospital units.[6] Many patients will respond to standard ACLS resuscitation, including high-quality CPR and rapid defibrillation. Rapid defibrillation (within 1 minute) is associated with survival to hospital discharge rates as high as 100% in this population.[7] A subset of patients who develop cardiac arrest during PCI will require prolonged resuscitation efforts. Providing effective prolonged resuscitation in the catheterization laboratory has unique challenges, and a number of interventions and adjuncts for management of cardiac arrest during PCI have been described. Inconsistent availability and lack of comparative studies limit recommendations of one approach over another. The 2015 ILCOR systematic review addressed the question of whether any special interventions or changes in care, compared with standard ACLS resuscitation alone, can improve outcomes in patients who develop cardiac arrest during PCI. There are a number of mechanical devices available to provide hemodynamic support during cardiac catheterization in high-risk patients presenting with cardiogenic shock. The use of these devices in cardiogenic shock was not reviewed by ILCOR in 2015. Therefore, the 2015 AHA Guidelines Update for CPR and ECC does not make recommendations on the use of mechanical support devices in patients presenting in cardiogenic shock who undergo PCI. Recent recommendations for the use of mechanical support devices in these situations can be found in the 2013 American College of Cardiology Foundation (ACCF)/AHA Guideline for the Management of ST-Elevation Myocardial Infarction.[8]

2015 Evidence Summary

The feasibility of using mechanical CPR devices during PCI has been demonstrated in both animal[9] and human[10–13] studies. No comparative studies have examined the use of mechanical CPR devices compared with manual chest compressions during PCI procedures. However, a number of case reports[9,10,14] and case series[12,13] have reported the use of mechanical CPR devices to facilitate prolonged resuscitation in patients who have a cardiac arrest during PCI. One study demonstrated that the use of a mechanical CPR device for cardiac arrest during PCI was feasible; however, no patients survived to hospital discharge.[12] Other studies have reported good patient outcomes, including ROSC, survival to discharge, and functional outcome at hospital discharge, after use of mechanical devices in resuscitation from cardiac arrest during PCI.[9,13] Mechanical CPR devices may also allow the use of fluoroscopy during chest compressions without direct irradiation of personnel. Patients in cardiogenic shock or with other high-risk features (e.g. multivessel coronary disease) may be at increased risk for adverse outcomes during or after PCI. Ventricular assist devices, intraaortic balloon pumps (IABP), and ECPR are all rescue treatment options available to support circulation and permit completion of the PCI. Not all interventions are available or can be rapidly deployed in all centers.

Not all interventions are available or can be rapidly deployed in all centers.

Rapid initiation of ECPR or cardiopulmonary bypass is associated with good patient outcomes in patients with hemodynamic collapse and cardiac arrest in the catheterization lab.[15–21] The use of ECPR is also feasible and associated with good outcomes when used as a bridge to coronary artery bypass grafting.[15,21–23] The combination of ECPR and IABP has been associated with increased survival when compared with IABP alone for patients who present with cardiogenic shock, including those who have a cardiac arrest while undergoing PCI.[16,20,24] Available observational studies often implement ECPR 20 to 30 minutes after cardiac arrest.[16,18] IABP counterpulsation increases coronary perfusion, decreases myocardial oxygen demand, and improves hemodynamics in cardiogenic shock states, but it is not associated with improved patient survival in cardiogenic shock.[25–23] The role of IABP in patients who have a cardiac arrest in the catheterization laboratory is not known. Several case series have reported on the use of emergency coronary artery bypass graft surgery after failed PCI.[34,35] In patients with cardiogenic shock or cardiac arrest and failed PCI, mechanical CPR devices and/or ECPR have been used as rescue bridges to coronary artery bypass graft. Although no comparison studies have examined the use of this therapy as an adjunct to PCI, survival to hospital discharge rates as high as 64% have been reported.[15,16,21,23]

2015 Recommendations - New and Updated
ACLS Modifications It may be reasonable to use mechanical CPR devices to provide chest compressions to patients in cardiac arrest during PCI (Class IIb, LOE C-EO). It may be reasonable to use ECPR as a rescue treatment when initial therapy is failing for cardiac arrest that occurs during PCI (Class IIb, LOE C-LD). Because patients can remain on ECPR support for extended periods of time without possibility of recovery, practical and ethical considerations must be taken into account in determining which victims of cardiac arrest should receive ECPR support. Institutional guidelines should include the selection of appropriate candidates for use of mechanical support devices to ensure that these devices are used as a bridge to recovery, surgery or transplant, or other device (Class I, LOE C-EO). Due to a lack of comparative studies, it is not possible to recommend one approach (manual CPR, mechanical CPR, or ECPR) over another when options exist.

The Australian and New Zealand guidelines

These guidelines discuss the use of mechanical CPR in an arrest during PCI [6]. Interestingly, they also discuss cough CPR for which they found some case reports in electrophysiology labs. They discuss drainage of pericardial tamponade in an arrest or thoracotomy and pericardiotomy with a class B recommendation if pericardiocentesis fails. In their handbook, they also state that 'The Interventionalist is heavily task burdened and as such is seldom in a good position to lead the resuscitation, and that 'CPR is likely to be required and there may be some tension between this and the ability of the interventionalist to continue with the procedure', indicating an understanding of the particular challenges faced in a catheter lab.

Current Guidelines : European Resuscitation Council Guidelines 2021

The 2021 ERC guidelines make quite significant modifications both to its posters and to the catheter laboratory recommendations. The general algorithm poster is now as follows and of note there is also a specific recommendation for in hospital resuscitation.

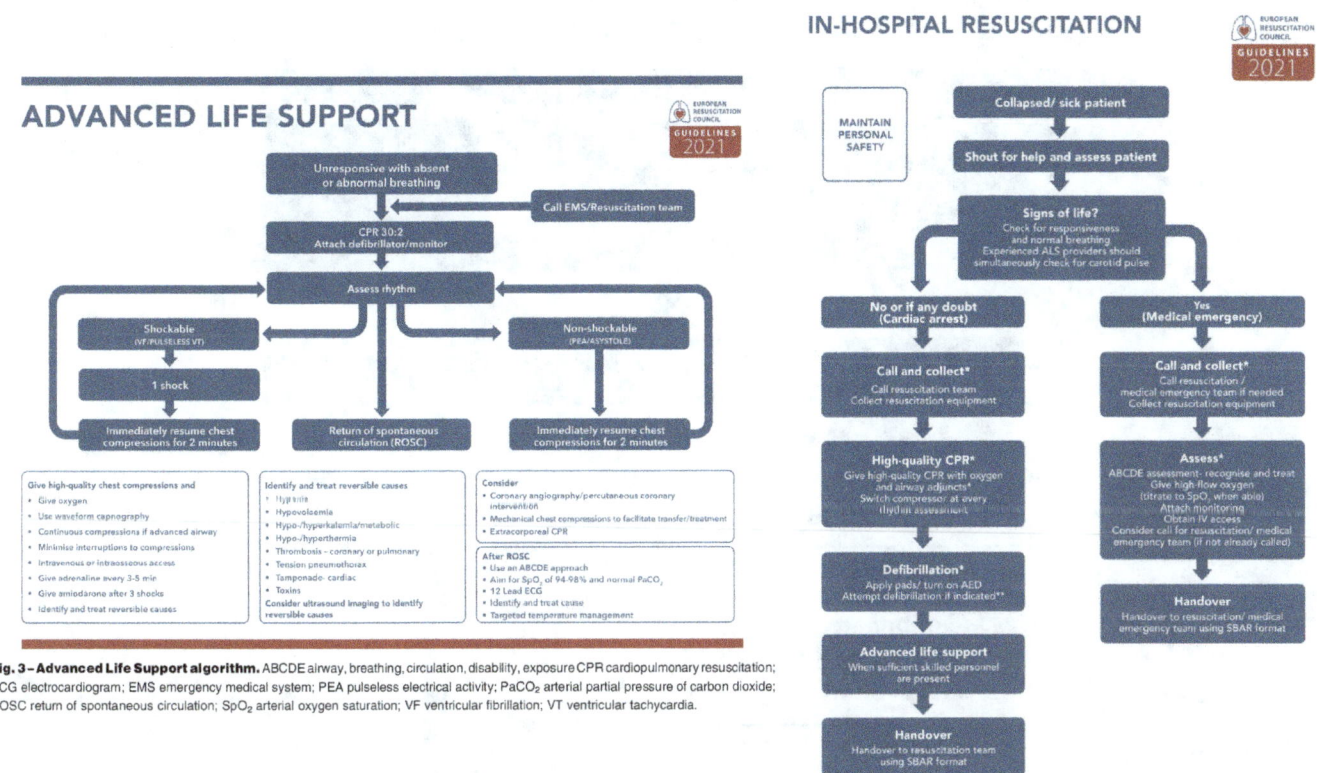

Fig. 3 – Advanced Life Support algorithm. ABCDE airway, breathing, circulation, disability, exposure CPR cardiopulmonary resuscitation; ECG electrocardiogram; EMS emergency medical system; PEA pulseless electrical activity; PaCO₂ arterial partial pressure of carbon dioxide; ROSC return of spontaneous circulation; SpO₂ arterial oxygen saturation; VF ventricular fibrillation; VT ventricular tachycardia.

The European Resuscitation Guidelines do also have a very comprehensive chapter on arrest in the catheter laboratory and a separate poster that they give for this area.

CARDIAC CATHETERISATION LABORATORY

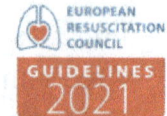

1. Prevent and be prepared
- Ensure adequate training of the staff in technical skills and ALS
- Ensure well-functioning and availability of equipment
- Use safety checklists

2. Detect cardiac arrest and activate cardiac arrest protocol
- Check patient's status and monitored vital signs regularly
- Consider cardiac echocardiogram in case of haemodynamic instability or suspected complication
- Shout for help and activate cardiac arrest protocol

3. Resuscitate and treat possible causes

VF / pVT cardiac arrest

Asystole / PEA

Defibrillate
(apply up to 3 consecutive shocks)

No ROSC

- Resuscitate according to **ALS algorithm**
- Check and correct potentially reversible causes including echocardiography and angiography
- Consider mechanical chest compression and circulatory support devices (including extracorporeal-CPR)

Catheterisation laboratory

The type of patients treated and procedures performed in the catheterisation laboratory has evolved over the last years towards greater complexity. More critically ill patients now undergo percutaneous coronary intervention (PCI) or implant of ventricular assist devices, and the volume of structural heart interventions, mostly offered to high-risk patients who are unfit for surgery, is rapidly increasing (i.e. percutaneous valve replacement or repair, leaks, septal defects or left atrial appendage closure). As a result, cardiac arrest in the catheterisation laboratory may occur in critically ill patients (i.e. cardiogenic shock due to extensive myocardial infarction), but also in stable patients undergoing planned procedures, which carry inherent potential hazards and are extremely sensitive to both technical and human factors.

Updated robust data on the global incidence of cardiac arrest in the catheterisation laboratory are lacking; registries mostly refer to PCI and show incidence rates highly dependent on patient pre-procedural risk.[433,434]

Evidence based recommendations derive from the ILCOR CoSTR documents[238,435,436] and ILCOR systematic reviews,[273] expert consensus statements from the European Association of Percutaneous Cardiovascular Interventions (EAPCI),[437] the Society for Cardiovascular Angiography and Interventions (SCAI),[438] and the International ECMO Network and The Extracorporeal Life Support Organization (ELSO),[439] plus focused literature search for evidence update. Where insufficient quality of evidence was obtained, recommendations were established by consensus expert within the writing group.

Prevent and be prepared

Ensure adequate training of the staff in technical skills and ALS
Staff working in the catheterisation laboratory should be adequately trained in resuscitation technical skills and ALS, including team and leadership training (Figs. 12 and S1).[435] Protocols for specific emergency procedures (e.g. initiation of mechanical CPR, emergency transcutaneous or transvenous pacing, pericardiocentesis, ventricular assist devices) should be established. On-site emergency drills should be considered to facilitate implementation and familiarisation of the staff.[438]

Ensure availability and well-functioning of emergency equipment
Emergency equipment should be clearly identified and the staff should be aware of its location to minimise delays if needed. Proper functioning should be regularly tested.

Use safety checklists
The use of safety checklists to minimise human factors should be encouraged,[437,438,440] since their use has been associated with fewer procedural complications and improved team communication.[441]

Detect cardiac arrest and activate cardiac arrest protocol

Check patient's status and monitored vital signs periodically
Continuous monitoring of vital signs (invasive blood pressure, heart rate and rhythm, pulse oximetry, capnography) facilitates early recognition and management of complications to prevent further deterioration and should be periodically checked. For example, high-degree atrioventricular block can occur during PCI, septal alcohol ablation or transaortic valve replacement (TAVR); chest pain, haemodynamic instability and ST-elevation in the ECG may be an alert for acute stent thrombosis during PCI or coronary ostium occlusion during TAVR; sudden hypotension requires ruling out pericardial tamponade (due to coronary perforation, atrial/ ventricular wall perforation or annulus rupture during balloon valvotomy or TAVR) or hypovolaemia in case of vascular complications. Defibrillation pads should be attached to at least all STEMI patients and considered in cases of complex PCI or high-risk patients.[438]

Consider cardiac echocardiography in case of haemodynamic instability or suspected complication
Cardiac echocardiography can help to detect complications and should rapidly be performed in case of haemodynamic instability. In procedures performed under transoesophageal echocardiography monitoring, this may provide better quality imaging for quicker and more precise identification of complications.[422]

Shout for help and activate cardiac arrest protocol
Once cardiac arrest is confirmed, the resuscitation team should be called immediately. Even if staff in the catheterisation laboratory should initiate resuscitation without delay, additional support may be required to allow on-going resuscitation while specific procedures to treat possible causes of arrest are performed (i.e. PCI, pericardiocentesis, invasive pacing). Leadership and roles during resuscitation should be clearly identified especially if new rescuers take over, to ensure coordinated and effective performance.

Resuscitate and treat possible causes

Resuscitate according to the modified ALS algorithm
Cardiac arrest in the catheterisation laboratory should be managed according to the ALS protocol, with some modifications.[101] In the presence of monitored VF/pVT, consider immediate defibrillation with up to three stacked shocks before starting chest compressions. In case of asystole/PEA, CPR and drugs should be administered according to the ALS protocol.

Check for reversible causes, including the use of echocardiography and angiography.

Identifying reversible causes is especially critical in non-shockable rhythms, for which cardiac echocardiography should be performed, and angiography considered if appropriate. Point of care ultrasonography (POCUS) can help to identify reversible causes of cardiac arrest, although attention should be paid to minimising pauses in chest compression.[442–444] In this regard, transoesophageal echocardiography may be helpful to enable continuous, higher-quality imaging assessment without interfering with resuscitation efforts.[445,446]

Consider mechanical compressions and percutaneous circulatory support devices
A Cochrane review including 11 trials comparing mechanical CPR versus manual chest compressions during CPR for adult patients suffering IHCA or OHCA arrest failed to prove superiority of mechanical over conventional CPR. However, the role of mechanical CPR was recognised as a reasonable alternative in settings where high-quality chest compressions are not possible or dangerous for the provider.[272] Delivering quality manual CPR in the catheterisation

laboratory may be challenging due to the presence of the X-ray tube, and may expose the rescuer harmful radiation; for this reason, mechanical CPR should be considered.

Percutaneous ventricular assist devices such as intra-aortic balloon pump, Impella® [447] or TandemHeart® may provide circulatory support while performing rescue procedures during cardiac arrest, although their use in this setting has not been extensively evaluated. Veno-arterial extracorporeal membrane oxygenation (VA-ECMO) offers both circulatory and pulmonary support and may be used in cardiac arrest (extracorporeal life support: ECPR), but there is insufficient evidence to systematically recommend such strategy.[238] A recent systematic review comparing ECPR to manual or mechanical CPR reported positive outcomes of ECPR in seven studies assessing their use for adult IHCA, although these were handicapped by their observational nature and limited internal validity.[273] Other smaller series have reported successful use of ECPR for in-hospital refractory cardiac arrest due to acute myocardial infarction[448] or complicating PCI or TAVR.[449] Should ECPR be considered, rapid initiation rather than waiting for complete failure of conventional measures is recommended,[439,450] since shorter conventional CPR (low-flow) time is a key factor for success.[451] Until randomised trials provide more consistent evidence, decisions to use ECPR or other ventricular assist devices should be adapted to the case, availability and expertise of the team.

Dialysis unit

ERC guidelines

These guidelines now specifically recommend that all staff in catheter laboratories have training in Mechanical CPR devices emergency pacing protocols and on site drills in catheter laboratories. It recommends checklists in the same way that we recommend the flipcharts in catheter laboratories and it recommends echocardiography as a routine part of the resuscitation.

Thus these guidelines have been very supportive of the concepts of the REACT guidelines.

Identification of the arrest and categorising the rhythm

We are able to identify the arrest much more quickly in order to get started with the resuscitation protocol. There is no need to look listen and feel for 10 seconds for a patient whose arterial blood pressure is being transduced and displayed, and whose continuous ECG monitoring is in clear view. We can also immediately determine the arrest rhythm, and we feel that due to this, there is benefit in separating the protocol into the 3 streams of VF or pulseless VT, Asystole, and PEA rather than the 2 streams of the universal algorithm.

The cardiac arrest will almost always be immediately identified. In Ventricular Fibrillation there is no other explanation for that ECG appearance and a member of the team should call out that there is a cardiac arrest. It would be most ideal if this was the cardiologist and they followed it up by any suspicions they have as to the cause. For example 'We have gone into Ventricular Fibrillation, this is a cardiac arrest. I just poked the wire into the ventricle doing this pacemaker, that must of caused it', or 'Cardiac Arrest, this is ventricular fibrillation. I think the LAD stent just blocked off a diagonal vessel'. This immediately tells the team what the cardiologist is thinking and potentially what interventions might be needed to resolve the situation.

The second rhythm that may occur is asystole. Again this cannot be mistaken and should immediately trigger the cardiac arrest call. There is no need to check for lead disconnection as for many years now the trace disappears from the screen if there is a lead disconnection.

The third category of Pulseless Electrical Activity can sometimes be less straightforward to diagnose. PEA means any ECG trace that could potentially support a cardiac output, so the QRS complexes can be narrow or wide. The diagnosis is made much more straightforward if the arterial trace is being transduced. If the arterial trace is non pulsetile then that patient has most likely arrested and if the sats trace is also non pulsetile then this becomes a certainty as this is an independent monitor.

There are two further caveats here, in that Ventricular Tachycardia can have a pulse or not have a pulse and also must not be mistaken for PEA. Thus any regular looking rhythm which looks to have a rate above 140 should be diagnosed as pulseless VT if the arterial trace is non-pulsetile. Furthermore extreme bradycardia, by which we mean less than 30 beats per minute, we have placed in the same group as asystole as it may respond to pacing. Thus in summary PEA needs to have a rate of above 30 and less than 140. Damn ! It suddenly got complicated. But this is all in a good cause as we want to be able to shock rapidly any rhythms that might be resuscitated with defibrillation, and we want to be able to pace any very slow rhythms that might respond to pacing. PEA is really the leftover category that is not amendable to electrical intervention.

Finally we should mention cases where the arterial trace is not being transduced such as pacing or even left atrial ablation cases. VF and Asystole is easy but if you have PEA or VT or extreme bradycardia then this situation does require 10 seconds of look listening and feeling. Absence of a pulse and motionlessness from the patient diagnoses a cardiac arrest.

At this point we should perhaps mention that we think that all people coming into an arrest in the cath lab should wear lead aprons. There is often a temptation to rush in unprotected in an emergency but all too often in that emergency, one person will get heavily involved in a task and then before they know it the cardiologist is taking long fluoroscopy images to try to open an occluded vessel.

Another departure in our protocol is that the general algorithm calls the arrest team, commences external cardiac massage and then assesses the rhythm. We recommend the exact opposite. We recommend assessing the rhythm as it is immediately available on the monitor, we don't recommend massage until after defibrillation, and percussion pacing rather than massage for asystole while the external pacing is set up, and we do not recommend calling the arrest team until we have a well-established cardiac arrest that has not responded to our initial urgent interventions and only if particular gaps in our staff mix are identified that need to be filled like an anaesthetist.

Ventricular fibrillation or pulseless VT

If the rhythm is ventricular fibrillation or pulseless VT then we do not recommend external cardiac massage but instead we recommend immediately placing the pads on the patient and giving 3 stacked shocks. This is quite a significant departure from recommended guidelines as commencing CPR as soon as an arrest is identified or even suspected is a cornerstone of the universal algorithm. But we recommend this pause in CPR for two reasons. Firstly there have been no studies ever produced that have demonstrated a survival benefit or increased likelihood of the defibrillation working after external cardiac massage in the first few minutes of the arrest.[36] The benefit comes later or in prolonged arrests, and therefore as our arrest is immediately identified then the priority should be to administer defibrillation as soon as possible, and as every catheter lab has a defibrillator either in the lab or very nearby this should be possible within 20-30 seconds of identifying the arrest.

The second reason for recommending a delay is that there are many reports documenting the trauma caused by CPR. In a systematic review performed in 2014, in addition to a 30% rate of rib fractures, there was a 2% flail chest rate, the possibility of coronary laceration, a 2% incidence of aortic laceration or dissection and the possibility of air embolism.[37]

It is also for this reason that we do not recommend following the universal algorithm's recommendation of compressing the chest to between 5 and 6cm. For those patients with an arterial trace being transduced, we recommend that you can titrate your external cardiac massage to achieve a systolic of 60mmHg. This would most often allow more gentle external compressions to safely be performed. However on occasion it might also allow the diagnosis of tamponade. This is because if you are unable to achieve a good systolic impulse when the arterial trace is being transduced no matter how hard you compress the chest, this can usually only be due to a mechanical cause - either tamponade meaning that the heart is compressed already by blood so that it cannot fill as you release the compressions, or extreme hypovolaemia (ie severe bleeding) whereby it is too empty to eject on compression.

Administering 3 stacked shocks is our preferred algorithm and is supported by the European Resuscitation council. In fact the reason that the universal algorithm was changed away from 3 stacked shocks for all patients in 2010 was due to the fact that when patients collapse out of hospital or in ward situations in hospitals, there is often a significant delay to the identification of the arrest, during which time the heart becomes distended. This was leading to patients who were successfully cardioverted, not regaining a spontaneous circulation as the heart was too distended to generate a reasonable blood pressure. This logic is irrelevant in the cath lab and in all situations whereby the arrest is identified immediately. We are of the view that the advantage of 3 stacked shocks probably only holds for the first cycle of resuscitation which is the reason that after the first cycle we recommend returning to single shocks with immediate massage. The chance of these subsequent shocks succeeding is much reduced and priority is now given to delivering good external cardiac massage while other interventions attempt to rescue the patient. We do not recommend a precordial thump, even though it is a potentially successful intervention. The reason for this is that with a defibrillator very close to hand in every catheter lab, this is much more likely to work and there is unlikely to be a significant delay between the opportunity to perform a precordial thump and the opportunity to defibrillate the patient, together with the lessened risk of trauma to the patient with electrical energy.

Asystole or extreme bradycardia

As with an arrest in VF, we do not recommend commencing external cardiac massage if asystole is identified. We recommend that you attach the pads (Which may already have been placed as a safety step for elective patients), but importantly ECG leads must be attached to the patient and then the pacing menu opened. The pacing is also started by default at a low amplitude and this must be turned up quickly. Our addition of extreme bradycardia to the asystole category is perhaps a little unusual but as it may also be remedied by external pacing leading to a return of spontaneous circulation it was felt that this may be a potential benefit with little chance of harm or confusion.

Pulseless Electrical activity, the H's and the T's.

As already mentioned we have split the identification of the rhythm back into 3 categories in order to make sure that the greatest number of patients possible might benefit from either defibrillation or external pacing. This does leave the category of patients with pulseless electrical activity seemingly without a straightforward intervention to benefit them. However the reason that the heart maintains its rhythm but the blood pressure disappears is often because the cause of the PEA arrest is not intrinsically due to an abnormality with the heart such as ischaemia or heart block. A common cause in the catheter lab might be a tamponade and an alternative might be severe hypovolaemia or anaphylaxis with vasodilation. Therefore in these patients, efforts may be directed towards searching for these causes. The General algorithm called these the H's and the T's, however there is a more limited range of these in the catheter lab to consider and thus we have not placed these specifically in the protocol, and the reason can be seen if we consider them one by one.

Hypoxia – we have an airway and breathing protocol with a person allocated to address this in an arrest.

Hypovolaemia - bleeding. We do specifically suggest considering the 4 common areas for bleeding in the cath lab – Haemothorax, Retroperitoneal or vascular Bleed, Aortic Dissection and Tamponade. Hypo/Hyperkalaemia, H+ Ion imbalance and electrolyte abnormalities are addressed by our recommendation to perform an early blood gas. It would be unusual for a patient in the cath lab to arrest from one of these as a primary cause in the cath lab, rather than acidosis being identified during a prolonged arrest.

Hypothermia is again unusual in a catheter lab, other than someone brought from an out of hospital arrest situation.

Tension pneumothorax – This is again part of our airway and breathing check allocated to role 2.

Tamponade – as this is high risk the recommendation for an early echocardiogram, the recommendations with regard to raising a concern over this if you cannot massage the patient to a systolic of 60mmHg, and our need to recommend treatment, we have actually promoted the importance of this above the standard H's and Ts.

Toxins – This would classically be an iatrogenic drug error in a cath lab, or much less likely an out of hospital arrest being brought to the cath lab in error. Any syringe drivers or infusions should be stopped in an arrest to address the possibility of a drug error.

Thrombosis-coronary or pulmonary – in catheter labs this would mean coronary occlusion with would most typically be due to a PCI or complication of this and therefore is again uppermost in our minds in our arrests. Pulmonary Emboli causing an arrest is less common especially due to our high use of antiplatelets and anticoagulants but it is prudent to maintain a high level of suspicion with regard to this. In an arrest it is very difficult to diagnose but in the periarrest situation, an echo showing right ventricular distension and failure in a disproportionate amount compared to the left ventricle that might look underfilled, would make the diagnosis likely. We ask for this to be considered in our protocol.

Adrenaline, Amiodarone, and Automated CPR devices

Due to the importance of Mechanical CPR we recommend that this is placed after only one cycle of manual CPR. This is because it is not recommended to perform any PCI with manual CPR due to the risk of the rescuer and it is not adviseable to have long periods without CPR and thus the Mechanical CPR device is the only solution to prolonged arrests.

Our algorithm recommends the administration of Adrenaline 1mg after the 3rd cycle and every other cycle thereafter. In addition Amiodarone is recommended at the same time, and it is at this stage that the arrest is becoming established and all easily reversible causes may have already been attempted. In addition this might support the patient until extracorporeal CPR can be set up if it is available. Where available, this can support the patients for a much longer period of time while the aetiology of the arrest is further investigated.

Special Circumstances

We have an area of the protocol dedicated to reminding us of the possible options in a series of specific arrest scenarios.

PCI – An arrest in a non-emergency PCI procedure is most likely to be due to the results of the intervention on the coronary arteries. There may be ischaemia secondary to vessel or side-branch occlusion, or hyperacute stent occlusion, or vessel dissection or perforation. The key to this arrest is most often to allow the cardiologist the time to attempt to resolve the situation interventionally, most often by means of a covered stent. This will require the cardiologist to have an assistant and also perhaps an unscrubbed assistant who can concentrate on the equipment needed and not get involved in the management of the arrest itself. It will also take coordination between the cardiologist and the external cardiac massage to allow him to perform the intervention. Pericardiocentesis may also be required if there is a perforated vessel. In terms of resources, it will also be important to consider emergency surgery in appropriate patients although this is becoming much rarer than in the past.

An IABP is a controversial topic now after the SHOCK-II trial failed to prove a definite benefit over its randomised control arm, the use of the IABP in the acutely unwell patient is becoming less common.

We have recommended one minute pauses for intervention although uninterrupted massage with an automated compression device while performing angiography is most likely preferable if it is available and we recommend that an automated CPR device should always be available to all teams.

Pacemakers and Ablations – the major risk of these interventions is for Tamponade. This should be suspected and echocardiography should be performed early. Pericardiocentesis should also be performed with Echo guidance, and should only be performed by an experienced practitioner who had done it many times in the non-arrest situation.

TAVI – It is in fact remarkable how safe modern TAVI has become, but many potential complications can still occur. Ostial obstruction is often a concern, and sometimes a wire is placed in the left main stem as a safety step in case an urgent stenting procedure is required should the ostium be inadvertently covered. If the patient arrests and ostial occlusion is suspected but it is not possible to stent it back open, it is also possible to grasp the TAVI valve and pull it back into the ascending aorta to allow reperfusion. Inadvertent displacement of the valve would most commonly be over the ostia and again, if incorrectly placed, it is not possible to retrieve the Valve fully, but if it is suspected to have resulted in an arrest, pulling it back into the ascending aorta may resolve the situation. Occasionally an aortic annulus rupture is seen after a TAVI procedure. This may cause a tamponade requiring pericardiocentesis. However the next step is often to keep the patient quite hypotensive, often also intubated and ventilated, in order to prevent further bleeding. This is usually not a complication that a cardiac surgeon would consider feasible to repair operatively, and thus hypotensive management is the management of choice.

Pulmonary Embolus – We have placed this in the special circumstances section in order to remind people of its possibility. A PEA arrest, perhaps going in and out of arrest, with a distended right ventricle may alert the team to this possibility. If the patient has arrested due to pulmonary embolus then thrombolysis might be the ideal treatment. If the patient has a pulse, immediate thrombolysis even prior to transfer to a CT scanner for confirmation may be safest if they are very unstable. Also surgical pulmonary embolectomy should be considered in very unstable patients as they will be placed on cardiopulmonary bypass and therefore there will be some time to stabilise the heart while the thrombi are removed.

Capnography in cardiac arrest

It is recommended that capnography is performed for patients in established cardiac arrest. Not only does this prove that the airways is patent and they have reasonable air entry to allow the exchange of CO_2, but more importantly the level of CO_2 exhaled by the lungs directly correlates with the cardiac output. If the CO_2 diminishes then tissue perfusion is reducing. In fact it is a good indicator of the quality of the resuscitation and in a more prolonged arrest, an end tidal CO_2 more than 20mmHg is a good prognostic indicator whereas an end tidal CO_2 of less than 10mmHg indicates a poor prognosis and may be used to indicate that further treatment is likely to be futile.

Return of Spontaneous Circulation

Congratulations if you successfully regain a perfusing rhythm. Regaining circulation means that the patient now has a lot more options and you have much more time to work out what has happened, but this is not the time to sit back and relax. The team now urgently need to investigate the cause and treat it quickly while the patient has a perfusing rhythm. A full ABC examination should be performed. Angiography should be performed, and also an echocardiogram by an experienced echocardiographer. If the patient has not recovered their GCS or still has hypoxia it is often safer to intubate them and ventilate them for a while rather than risk the hypoxia causing further arrests. It would also allow good vascular access with an arterial line, and central line and urinary catheter to allow cardiac monitoring and inotropes or vasoconstrictors as appropriate, and the appropriate intensive care area will have to be identified. If there has been a prolonged period of arrest then targeted temperature management with hypothermia for 24-48 hours has been proven to improve neurological outcome in out of hospital arrests and therefore may help a patient who has arrested for 20 minutes or more in hospital although there have been no in hospital studies to demonstrate the same benefit.

Cardiac Arrest in the Recovery area

It is important to note that the specialist protocol highlighted above is strictly for use in the catheter lab. Once the patient is in the recovery area then the ALS algorithm should be followed. Confusion over this could be life threatening as there could be confusion amongst staff as to whether we are pursuing a 3 shock protocol or one shock and straight onto massage protocol. If the person performing CPR was going straight back to massage as per the ALS guidelines but the person on the defibrillator was following REACT and delivering a shock for a second time, this could result in a critical event for the person delivering CPR as they could receive that shock. In addition it is not possible to perform fluoroscopy, we cannot perform PCI and the cardiologist will not be there for echocardiography, and we must call the cardiac arrest team as the REACT team are likely to be busy with patients in the catheter labs and we cannot assume that large numbers of people can immediately come to the recovery area from the cath labs.

However practice in this area can lead to improvements in outcomes when this occurs. Minor amendments to the arrest protocol would be to immediately seek help from the operating cardiologist, to bring an echo machine to the bedside to look for tamponade, to consider an automated CPR device and to consider returning the arrested patient back to a catheter lab to see if there has been a vessel occlusion for PCI, or a TAVI displacement. Finally in centres with the facility to apply extracorporeal CPR this could be considered here also, as the patient will have already been carefully assessed and treated and a cardiologist would be able to determine whether a period of extracorporeal CPR might be able to salvage the situation.

Acute Emergency Protocols

We have now dealt with the arrest situations in the catheter lab and have described in detail our protocols for that situation but in fact it is much more common for the catheter lab team to be facing an evolving acute emergency of the gradually deteriorating patient than an unheralded cardiac arrest. And thus we devote half of our course and the handbook to identification, management and investigation of acute emergencies in the catheter lab and also for acute emergencies in the recovery area. We believe that prompt treatment of these emergencies will in fact lead to rarer cardiac arrests and as there are a much greater range of therapies available when the patient has a pulse, early identification of the acute emergency is far preferable to treatment once arrested.

Hypotension and Arrhythmias

'These are only 3 causes of a low blood pressure'

Hypotension is the most common emergency both in the catheter lab and also in the recovery areas and wards. Prompt treatment – without waiting for definitive tests – can keep the patient alive while help or results are awaited. The underlying problems may be multifactorial: constant reassessment of one cause of hypotension may uncover another, thus, reassessment is mandatory.

A simple way of approaching hypotension is to consider the blood pressure as requiring 3 factors. A good blood supply to the heart (pre-load), good heart contractility (cardiac output) and a decent resistance in the arterial system, (after-load). After establishing whether the problem is before the heart, after the heart or a problem with the heart, it is possible to refine your diagnosis with further investigation. This is the reason that we say that there are only 3 causes of a low blood pressure. We consider arrhythmias separately as you usually notice the pulse or ECG before the blood pressure in those cases.

The five-point plan

We believe that the 5-point plan is crucial to a systemic method for approaching the patient but even more importantly for communicating this to your colleagues.

How often have you been frustrated by a clinician to whom you have asked advice and they have come up, had a poke at a few of the monitors and a bit of a read of the charts and then just recommended some fluids and walked off? While this may be the right course of action in that person's mind, they have not convinced you that they have made an adequate assessment, they have not told you what diagnosis is that they are treating, they have not told you the reason for that treatment and made no mention of any tests needed to confirm the diagnosis or a plan for review of the patient to make sure their plan is working.

Imagine instead a clinician who comes to your assistance, performs a quick but efficient assessment of the airway, the breathing and then the circulation including getting their stethoscope out to listen to the lungs and heart and a feel of the temperature of the patient. They then read the chart carefully and then say to you 'I think that this person has acute heart failure'. I recommend starting some dobutamine - 50mg in 50mls of saline at 5mls per hour. I think we should also check a blood gas, full blood count, electrolytes and a CXR. I will be back in 15 minutes to see how we are getting on, ring if you need me more urgently.

In actual fact both clinicians would probably take no more than a minute or two to enact the plans above but we should all strive to be that second clinician where we use a common language to communicate between us and a systematic approach to each patient.

The Five Point Plan

A structured approach to problems facilitates prompt and accurate diagnosis and treatment and active communication,

1. Assess

2. Diagnose

3. Action Plan

4. Investigate

5. Reassess

The 5-point plan asks you first to perform a comprehensive ABC assessment. Having a tension pneumothorax is a very embarrassing cause of a low blood pressure if you miss it!

Secondly the diagnosis is key. We must get in the habit in clearly communicating the diagnosis that we are working to. Once we have a diagnosis we can enact a plan to try to improve this situation. Of note Action comes before Investigations, you must do something to improve the patient clinically and only then do we move to investigations to check and support the diagnosis we are working towards.

And you must always communicate your timeframe for reassessment, even if it is just to come and soak up the praise for having done such a good job in fixing the patient! But if you haven't got it right or the patient's situation is changing then you need to pick it up early, not just when called again. This is proactive management rather than reactive patient management.

Assessment

Airway & Breathing

Turn oxygen up to 100% (even in COPD patients while you work out the problem)
If awake, check airway patency by talking to the patient. Use airway adjuncts if indicated.
Is the trachea central?
Look for bilateral chest movement and auscultate for air entry.
Specifically try to exclude a pneumothorax and a haemothorax every time you listen. (Also listen to the heart sounds while you have your stethoscope on the chest. Are the heart sounds muffled ? Is there a torrential systolic murmur?)
In a catheter lab with a patient on the table consider a single AP fluoroscopy view to exclude a large or tension pneumothorax, and to look for a big haemothorax (and to check for the size of the pericardial outline and size of aortic outline).

Circulation

Arterial line
If present, check the quality of the trace. Consider using a second arterial catheter transduction if you have double access.
If no arterial line, check carotid or femoral pulse and non-invasive blood pressure.
Also look at the quality of the Sats trace. If this is strong and the sats are normal this may indicate that there is a reasonable circulation, and equally if the trace is poor and not picking up it is further evidence of poor perfusion.

Central line or JVP
Check trace and if possible you might want to try to assess the JVP. This may be impossible if the patient is laid flat, but if reclined a little may be possible to see.

Other checks
Skin temperature
Capillary refill. Is this more than 5 seconds?
Is there a site for bleeding? Look at the puncture sites, assess the groin or abdomen for swelling or distension. Think about haemothorax or aortic dissection.

Diagnosis

Having performed a good clinical examination and assessed all immediately available parameters, make a "best guess" as to the clinical syndrome involved. If the patient is in extremis, treat immediately based on your best guess. The results of your intervention will either confirm or refute your diagnosis and allow you to make appropriate adjustments to your plan.

	Heart rate	Blood pressure	Arterial "swing"	JVP	Urine output	Peripheral temp	Capillary refill time (secs)
Hypovolaemia (e.g. bleeding, underfilled)	↑	↓	↑	↓↓	↓↓	↓	↑
Vasodilation (e.g. sepsis or anaphylaxis)	↑	↓		↓	↓	↑	↓
Low output state (e.g. tamponade or failure)	↑↑	↓		↑	↓	↓	↑
Arrhythmia (e.g. bradycardia or tachycardia)	↑↓	↓				↓	↑

The pattern of abnormalities gives clinical clues as to the underlying pathology. There may be some overlap in the signs and symptoms of different pathologies, but test interventions and investigations can help tease out the correct diagnosis.

Action Plan & Investigations

Your strategy should reflect the diagnosis you have made. Ensure that you vocalise your thoughts at this stage – team members can offer useful insight and informing them of the reasons for your management plan forewarns them of what else they may be required to do.

Once you have a Diagnosis, it is easy! Each syndrome comes with an Action Plan and then a set of investigations to confirm you are right!

Low Blood pressure.

We like to break down the causes of a low blood pressure down into 3 possibilities. We teach that there are in fact only 3 causes of a low blood pressure. The first and possibly most common is Hypovolaemia, a problem of a lack of filling of the heart. The second is vasodilation, or a problem with afterload of the heart and then finally a low output state which is a problem with the heart.

We like to consider a tachyarrhythmia and a bradyarrhythmia separately as usually we will notice the abnormal heart rate before any drop in blood pressure and addressing the heart rate will be the solution to resolving any hypotension in these patients.

Diagnosis: Hypovolaemia

The patient typically has a low blood pressure. There is a low JVP. The peripheries are cool and the capillary filling is prolonged. The patient may have a dry mouth and feel thirsty. The urine output may be low, with a small concentrated volume if the hypotension has led to reduced renal perfusion. If the cause of the low circulating volume is bleeding, You may be able to identify a distended abdomen or bruising or actual bleeding at the puncture site.

Action plan: Volume (colloid or blood)

    500ml colloid if the haemoglobin is maintained or blood if bleeding.

    Correct clotting abnormalities.

    If high volume blood loss, may need to make a plan to stop the bleeding :

    Puncture site bleeding : Compression, Femstop or vascular surgical repair.

    Retroperitoneal bleed : May require vascular surgery to address this perhaps after a
CT scan or Ultrasound.

    Haemothorax : Chest drain

    Aortic Dissection : This may require Thoracic Endovascular stenting or surgical treatment, or hypotensive management.

Investigations: ABG, fluoroscopy image of the chest (collection) , FBC, clotting, U&E.

    ABG may show falling Hb.

    CXR may show further blood in the chest with a haemothorax

    Clotting may be deranged and require correction or be normal

    Inform cardiologist of the action plan and the response to it by the patient

Diagnosis: Vasodilation (or anaphylaxis)

The patient has a low blood pressure, low or normal central venous pressure, warm peripheries, and a low urine output with a normal or even shortened capillary filling time. If the patient has had a fluid challenge, this often shows minimal response or a transient response.

Please note that you are guessing the diagnosis of vasodilation until you have an echo and an ECG. Always ask yourself, 'Am I missing a low output state'.

Also if the patient is also wheezy, or has a rash or widespread erythema then this may be an anaphylactic response to a drug such as the contrast media.

Action plan: Give 500mls of a colloid or crystalloid.
                      Adrenaline 0.5mls im of 1 in 1000 in the middle 1/3rd of the Thigh.
                      Or Metaraminol 1ml bolus of 10mg/ml diluted up to 10mls in normal
                      saline.
                      Or dobutamine 5mls per hour of 50mg in 50mls of normal saline as a
                      peripheral iv infusion.
                      If anaphylaxis suspected then give Hydrocortisone 200mg im or slow iv
                      If anaphylaxis suspected then give Chlorphenamine 50mg im or slow iv.
                      Inform cardiologist of the situation and the drugs given.

Investigations: 1. ABG, Fluoroscopy image of the chest, FBC, clotting, U&E.
                      2. ECG, Echocardiogram. Possibly a left ventriculogram.

The Echocardiogram will be the key to excluding the low output state, and the heart should be hyperdynamic. The valves should also be assessed, as a hyperdynamic heart with mitral papillary rupture and torrential Mitral regurgitation is a low output state.

An ECG should be checked just to give further evidence that there is no ischaemia, although the echocardiogram would also see a regional wall abnormality.

If PCI is being performed it may be easily possible to cross the aortic valve and do a left ventriculogram to assess the LV function rapidly

PA catheter (or other form of cardiac output monitoring) could help to confirm the diagnosis and also gives guidance on the doses of vasoconstrictor but this would most commonly only be placed in an intensive care unit

In the case of suspected anaphylaxis in addition to adrenaline, chlorphenamine and hydrocortisone, particular attention must be paid to protection of the airway and bronchoconstriction. If there is stridor, airway swelling, or desaturation below 93% then an anaesthetist must be called, 100% oxygen given via a non-rebreathing mask and the airway trolley brought to the catheter lab.

Diagnosis: Low Output state

The patient has a low blood pressure, a high JVP pressure, cold peripheries, prolonged capillary filling and low urine output, This may indicate a low output state. If assessment occurs after a fluid challenge, this may show worsening hypotension following fluid. While there may be several causes of a low output state including Tamponade, Myocardial Ischaemia or Infarction,

Valve dysfunction or just left ventricular failure, the initial management will be the same.

Action plan: Cardiac support with Dobutamine 5ml/hr of 50mg in 50mls of normal
                    saline via a peripheral iv cannula.
                    Or Metaraminol 1ml bolus of 10mg/ml diluted up to 10mls in normal
                    saline.
                    Consider an IABP as further supportive measure.

Investigations: 1. ABG, fluoroscopy image (globular heart) , FBC, clotting, U&E,
                    2. ECG, Echocardiogram. Angiogram and Possibly a left
                    ventriculogram.
                    Fluoroscopy may show widened mediastinum or globular heart.
                    ECG may indicate ischaemia.
                    Echocardiogram may show pericardial effusion and tamponade, valve
                    failure or poor contractility. A distended right ventricle would also alert
                    us to the possibility of a pulmonary embolus.
                    A Left ventriculogram may show a poorly functioning left ventricle to
                    secure the diagnosis of a low output state, and an angiogram may
                    demonstrate an occluded or dissected vessel or stent.

After further investigation and diagnosis :

Tamponade	-requires pericardiocentesis and to address the cause of the bleed.
Left ventricular failure	- requires increasing inotropic support +/- IABP.
Valve failure	- may require surgical repair
Ischaemia/infarction	- requires revascularisation.
Pulmonary Embolus	- Thrombolysis.

Arrhythmias

A structured approach to arrhythmias helps to instigate prompt treatment. Bedside monitoring is useful for making initial plans for treatment, although a 12-lead ECG further delineates the exact underlying problem. It is useful to know if the arrhythmia is fast or slow, regular or irregular, with broad or narrow complexes.

	Rate	Irregular	Broad	Other
Atrial fibrillation (AF)	↑	Y	N	Patient rarely loses consciousness.
Supraventricular tachycardia (SVT)	↑	N	N	P waves absent or abnormal. Patient rarely loses consciousness.
Ventricular tachycardia (VT)	↑	N	Y	Patient may well lose consciousness.
Sinus tachycardia	↑	N	N	With P-waves.
Sinus bradycardia	↓	N	N	
Nodal or junctional rhythm	↑↓	N	N	P waves absent or abnormal.

Diagnosis; Fast Rhythm (Tachyarrhythmia)

The most important distinction to make between the various fast rhythms is whether they are haemodynamically stable or not. Atrial Fibrillation (AF), Supraventricular tachyarrhythmia (SVT), or Ventricular tachyarrhythmia (VT) will present with normal or low blood pressure, normal or low JVP, cool peripheries and, frequently, low urine output. VT should raise a suspicion of ischaemia.

Action Plan: correct electrolytes, give colloid, optimize oxygenation
            $Mg2+$ 8mmol bolus
            K+ as per local protocol, usually 10 – 20mmol as slow infusion
            Hemodynamically stable- : amiodarone 300mg IV over 20 – 60 mins
            Hemodynamically unstable : synchronized DC cardioversion
            Consider amiodarone 300mg over 10-20min if 3 shocks fail

Investigations: 12 lead ECG, ABG, FBC, U&E
                           FBC may uncover signs of infection leading to sinus or other
                           tachycardia
                           ECG may suggest ischaemia prompting need for
                           revascularisation

Diagnosis: Slow rhythm (bradycardia)
                           The patient may be hypotensive with a low or normal CVP, cool
                           peripheries and a low urine output. Ask how they feel and if they
                           feel ill or dizzy.

Action plan: Atropine 600mcg bolus, repeated up to 3mg.
                           Isoprenaline 2mg in 50 ml of normal saline at 5mls per hour
                           OR adrenaline 5mg in 50ml starting at 5mls per hour.
                           if these both fail, consider external pacing or transvenous pacing.

Respiratory Emergencies

Patients with respiratory or airway problems frequently manifest with an immediately apparent circulatory problem. It is not uncommon, therefore, for practitioners to direct their attention to the circulation, glossing over examination of the airway and breathing and leaving this untreated. For this reason, it is particularly important to stress a systematic ABC approach.

The Five Point Plan

A structured approach to problems in the catheter lab or recovery area patient facilitates prompt and accurate diagnosis, prompts active communication and highlights the importance of frequent reassessment.

1. Assess

2. Diagnose

3. Action Plan

4. Investigate

5. Reassess

Assessment: Airway

Breathing patient

If the patient is talking to you, the airway is patent! Stridor or inability to talk, or gurgling upper airway sounds will alert you to a possible airway emergency.

Begin with 100% oxygen with a bag valve mask and also call for an anaesthetist. If the patient has a respiratory rate over 6 breaths per minute simply hold this securely over the patients nose and mouth. If they have reduced consciousness or reduced respiratory rate below 6 breaths per minute then you should perform a jaw thrust and chin lift and give additional breaths. If jaw thrust chin lift fails, and they are losing consciousness, attempt a guedel airway and use the bag valve mask. Check that the trachea is central and listen both sides for a pneumothorax or haemothorax, and for wheeze or crepitations.

An airway problem would most likely be airway occlusion due to reduced conscious level. It would be unlikely to be due to a foreign body in a catheter lab. The only other possibility would be due to upper airway oedema secondary to anaphylaxis. Either way for a breathing patient the protocol should be

> Airway and breathing protocol in a breathing patient
>> 100% Oxygen with a bag valve mask. – hold firmly over the face and let the patient breathe. Tell the cardiologist that you have an oxygenation problem and consider calling an anaesthetist.
>> If the saturations are still low, perform a jaw thrust/ chin lift and consider sup porting their own breathing with the bag or giving additional breaths.
>> If the saturations continue to be low and conscious level is dropping, consider guedel airway.
>> If there is still stridor or the possibility of an occluded airway, while waiting for an anaesthetist you could also consider a nasopharyngeal airway although this can cause bleeding or a laryngeal mask.
>> Always feel the trachea and listen both sides.
>>> For a pneumothorax – needle thoracentesis in the 2nd intercostal space (Below the second rib) followed by a drain. *
>>> If you hear crepitations – consider pulmonary oedema–Furosemide 40-80mg iv
>>> If you hear a wheeze – Salbutamol nebulisers.

> Investigations : May consider a blood gas and a fluoroscopy or portable CXR.

* Tension pneumothorax requires immediate decompression with a large bore venflon in the second intercostal space at the mid-clavicular line. Do not remove the metal needle as the plastic sheath will kink in the soft tissues and render this treatment useless. Of note the second inter-costal space is lower than some think and is below the rib joining the sterno-manubrial junction (angle of louis). If you really want to know if it was a tension pneumothorax, place water on the end of the venflon as you insert it and see if the water is blown out or sucked in.

A finger thoracostomy in the anterior axillary line in the 5th space (auscultatory triangle) is now regarded as a safer, and quicker alternative to the technique of a venflons in the 2nd intercostal space.

A chest drain must then be inserted as you have only converted a tension pneumothorax into a simple pneumothorax.

Non Breathing patient.

If the patient has lost consciousness and is not breathing then you must immediately activate the REACT emergency protocol, which will call an anaesthetist and get you help and you must assist the patient's breathing with a bag valve mask with oxygen at 100%. Perform a jaw thrust and chin lift and ensure you have a good seal with the mask. If you are have difficulty use two hands to create a good seal and get a second person to squeeze the bag. If the patient has a large beard then sleek tape can be used above and below the mouth to assist with obtaining a good seal.

Is there air entry and is the chest going up and down ? If there is then you can feel the trachea and listen to the chest to exclude a pneumothorax, haemothorax, wheeze and crepitations.

If you are not getting air entry then place a guedel airway and try the bag valve mask again.

If you are still not getting air entry then consider either a nasopharyngeal airway or a laryngeal mask. You could also consider asking for suction and try to perform suction to the back of the nasopharynx, but after attempting these 3 airway adjuncts and ensuring the airway is clear you are best to just continuing to perform 2 person Bag valve mask while awaiting the anaesthetist. You can also get the airway trolley and possibly the difficult airway trolley to the catheter lab.

The REACT Communication Board

REACT Communication Board

Name Age Consent	Cardiologist

Planned Procedure

Allergies	1. Emergency Leader
Medications	2. Airway and Breathing
Past History	3. Defibrillation/Pacing
Last Eaten	4. CPR
Events	5. Drugs and timing
LV function Rhythm Diabetes	6. Resource Coordinator
Blood tests Hb INR plts Cr	Available anaesthetist Contact number:
iv access	Available colleagues : Contact number:
Prior antiplatelets Prior anticoagulation	Anaesthetic issues
Antibiotic prophylaxis	G&S

In 2007 the WHO patient safety team launched 'safe surgery saves lives' and the WHO patient safety checklist was born a year later. In a large multinational, multicentre study, it was shown to reduce mortality and morbidity by increasing the adherence to accepted policies and guidelines. Over 10 years later, checklists are an integral part of patient safety across all interventional specialties. However one weakness of a checklist is that it does get tucked away in the notes after it has been completed and often they are not as tailored for the environment in which they are being used as they could be.

Thus while we understand and support the importance of getting together at the start of a session and also before each patient, we wanted to use the information gained in case of an emergency, and the only way to do this is to put it on the wall for the whole team to see!

Also it is important for this board to be full of only the important issues that will be useful to the team so we support local teams being able to modify their own boards to their particular needs. However we feel that the following information is important for emergency situations : Clearly name, age and gender is a good place to start on the board especially for people who come into an emergency and need to talk to the patient. Also the height and weight might be useful for some drug dosing and in the event of needing an IABP or eCPR.

Having the procedure clearly written on the board is vital for people coming in to try to help.

Having the AMPLE history on the board will again help in an emergency, so all clinicians know about allergies, and PMH and also if intubation is going to be necessary how likely aspiration might be due to stomach contents.

We feel that a key part of this board is to write down at the start of the day the people who would be fulfilling the 6 key roles in an emergency. This will provide the best clarity of all, if an emergency situation arises.

We recommend adding the locations of iv access, and whether antibiotics or antiplatelets have been used.

Then on the right hand side of the board there is an area to document in advance who will be in the REACT emergency if one is called. This may only need to be completed at the start of the day, although if someone goes on a break it might be good practice to change your name on the board before going to someone who will be present while you are away.

In addition to the REACT team, there is a section to document who the on call anaesthetist would be and their contact information, and also the name and contact details of a second anaesthetist. This may be an important piece of information and actually having the contact numbers on the board may save a significant amount of time.

Thus in summary we feel that as a WHO checklist is already being completed, that the addition of a communication board in every catheter lab would not significantly increase the time taken for a preoperative check and the added advantage of having all the important information easily visible and to hand will significantly help with any acute emergency or arrest. It will both help the team composition by the preallocation of roles and also help them to call any additional required personnel. Then if additional personnel come into the room that can use this board at a glance to obtain a rapid summary of the patients and the key issues regarding the patient.

The Emergency Flipcharts

We believe that an emergency is not the time to test your memory and that all emergencies including arrests, non-arrests in the catheter lab and emergencies in the recovery area should be planned for and the agreed protocols clearly written in an accessible format that can be read in the emergency. Therefore we have created a flipchart that includes important information that can be followed for each emergency that is encountered. We encourage clinicians to pick up the flipchart in every emergency and read it out in strong preference to trying to memorise it. We will go through each protocol in this section in some detail. The flipchart format is split into : actions that should be performed together with the dose recommendations for all drugs ; The people that may potentially be called for this emergency and the equipment that will be needed to address this situation.

The Cardiac Arrest Protocol

Actions
Allocate Emergency Leader with 6 key roles
100% O2, protect airway
VF – 3 stacked shocks at maximum amplitude
Asystole – Percussion pace, Externally pace 100bpm, then temporary wire
Adrenaline after 3rd CPR cycle, Then alternating cycles
Amiodarone after 3rd CPR cycle if VF
Exclude Pneumothorax /Haemothorax
Tamponade - Pericardiocentesis
Occlusion – PCI once mechanical CPR applied.
PE – Echo, thrombolysis, CT scan, Surgical Embolectomy
Consider Extracorporeal CPR

Cardiac Arrest

Follow REACT Protocol Poster

People	Equipment
Emergency Anaesthetist	Defibrillator with Pads
Call 2nd Cardiologist	Airway Trolley
Call CCU	Automated CPR device
Arrest team	Covered Stents
Notify ICU	Echocardiogram

In addition to the two posters for a cardiac arrest in the catheter lab, we have a flipchart sheet that may be read by the team leader. In the Actions column it documents some of the key interventions in the poster and in addition reminds the team leader to allocate the 6 key roles of his team immediately, followed by airway and breathing reminder to give 100% oxygen, and the protocol for the 3 rhythms of VF, asystole and PEA.

In the People column we recommend that an anaesthetist is immediately called and also a second cardiologist, and their contact numbers should be on the communication board. In addition the team leader should notify CCU and the ICU and then should consider calling the arrest team if the leader feels that they are short of staff or expertise in the room especially at night. The equipment needed will include a defibrillator, an airway trolley, and an automated CPR device. In addition there may be specific equipment needed according to the case, and for example a PCI case might need covered stents, and an echo and pericardiocentesis set might be needed in a tamponade.

The Cardiac Arrest Protocol

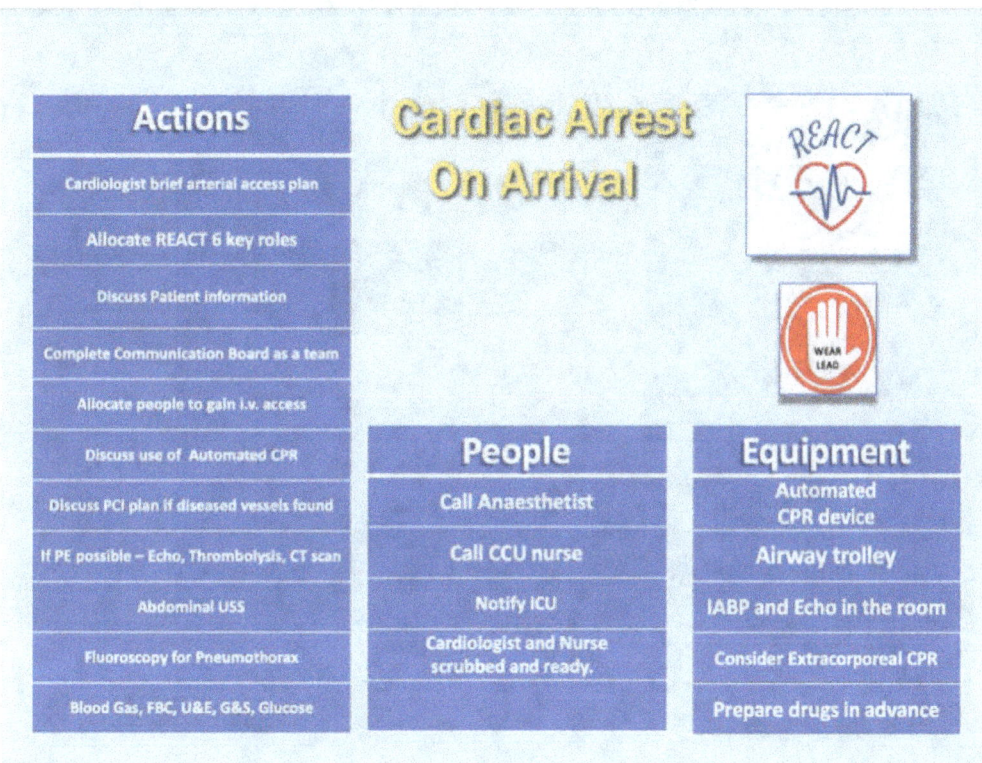

This is a sufficiently different scenario to the arrest of an elective patient to warrant its own protocol and specific practice for its occurrence. The REACT protocol can be followed but the flipchart provides an opportunity to more optimally prepare for this special situation.

If there has been a warning call from the location of the patient such as the Emergency department or the Ambulance then there is an opportunity for the team to get together and pre-allocate the REACT 6 key roles and also discuss the vascular and arterial access plan and the automated CPR device plan. Additional help can be sought including an anaesthetist and any additional help from the CCU. The communication board can be completed and the cardiologist and scrub nurse should be able to scrub ready for the patient to arrive.

If there is time then it is advisable to discuss the range of plans as widely as possible, including bloods that need to be taken, a PCI plan if there is coronary disease, a plan to do an echocardiogram if there is return of circulation, the plan if a pulmonary embolus is suspected, and possibly a plan for an abdominal ultrasound if no other cause for the arrest is found to exclude an abdominal aortic aneurysm rupture. It should perhaps be expected that the automated CPR device will be placed as soon as the patient is placed on the cath lab table.

Bleeding Emergency Protocol

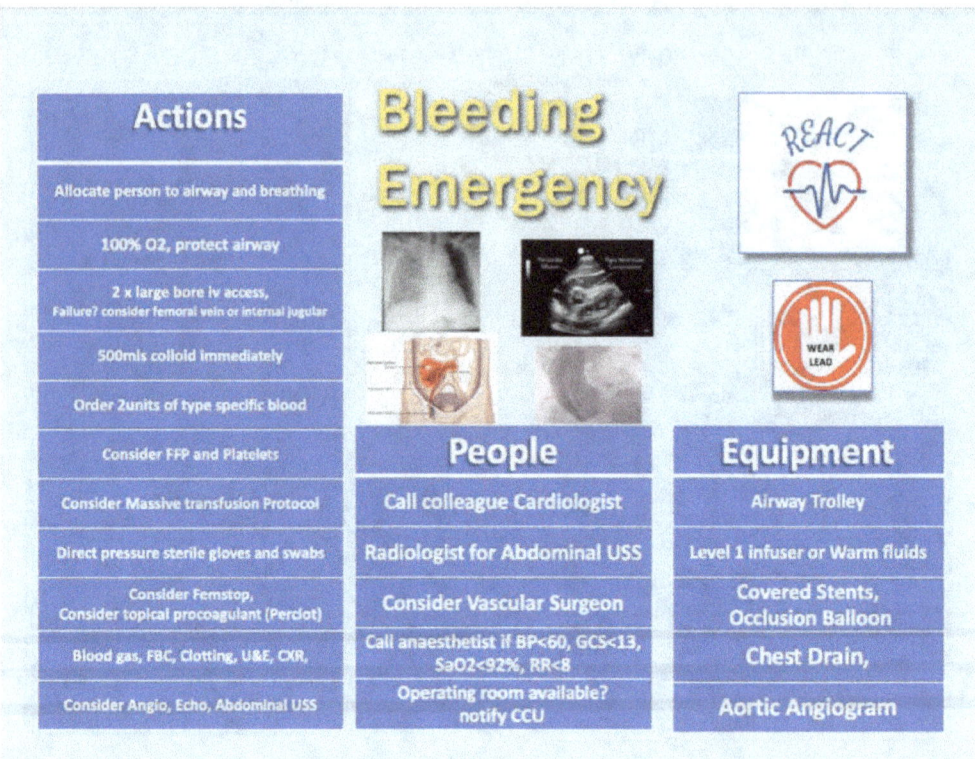

Either in the catheter lab or in the recovery room there is the possibility of a bleeding emergency. The possible locations of a bleed are from the arterial access site, the retroperitoneal space, a haemothorax, an aortic dissection or in the pericardium (Although blood in the pericardium would more commonly manifest as tamponade).

If this is suspected then anyone can activate the REACT protocol for this and the 6 key roles should be allocated. Importantly someone must go to the airway to make sure that it is protected and 100% oxygen given. Any obvious bleeding should be compressed. Then priority must be given to making sure there is adequate vascular access and the administration of colloid or blood. If there is clearly a bleed then many hospitals have a massive transfusion protocol and also access to Level 1 infusers that can administer warm blood or products quickly. Alternatively blood, FFP and platelets should be considered. Of note military resuscitation consists of 1:1 blood and FFP and in emergency departments, often a unit of FFP is given every 4 units of blood so remember to also consider clotting products.

We should seek help early, either to establish the diagnosis such as in a retroperitoneal bleed which may require an abdominal ultrasound performed by a radiologist, or if the bleed is clearly from access, then a vascular surgeon may be required. If there is a haemothorax then a chest drain would be required and then consideration of whether the subclavian vein or pulmonary vein has been injured. If there is a loss of blood pressure and the patient is cold and clammy then an aortic dissection should be considered and an aortic angiogram or echo performed and if an echo is performed a pericardial collection must be excluded.

If there has been a diagnosis of aortic dissection, despite this being a bleeding emergency it does need treating in a very different way. In contrast to keeping the blood pressure high and supporting with large volume fluids, the blood pressure should be kept much lower or even brought down lower with labetolol or via intubation and propofol. The higher the blood pressure the higher the risk that the aortic dissection will perforate through the adventitial layer of the aorta and the patient will become unsalvageable. In the situation of aortic dissection either a cardiac surgeon should be called to request emergency dissection repair or if the patient is not fit enough for this then vascular radiology may occasionally be able to place a TEVAR (Thoracic Endovascular Aortic Replacement stent) depending on the location of the aortic tear.

Vasodilation or anaphylaxis

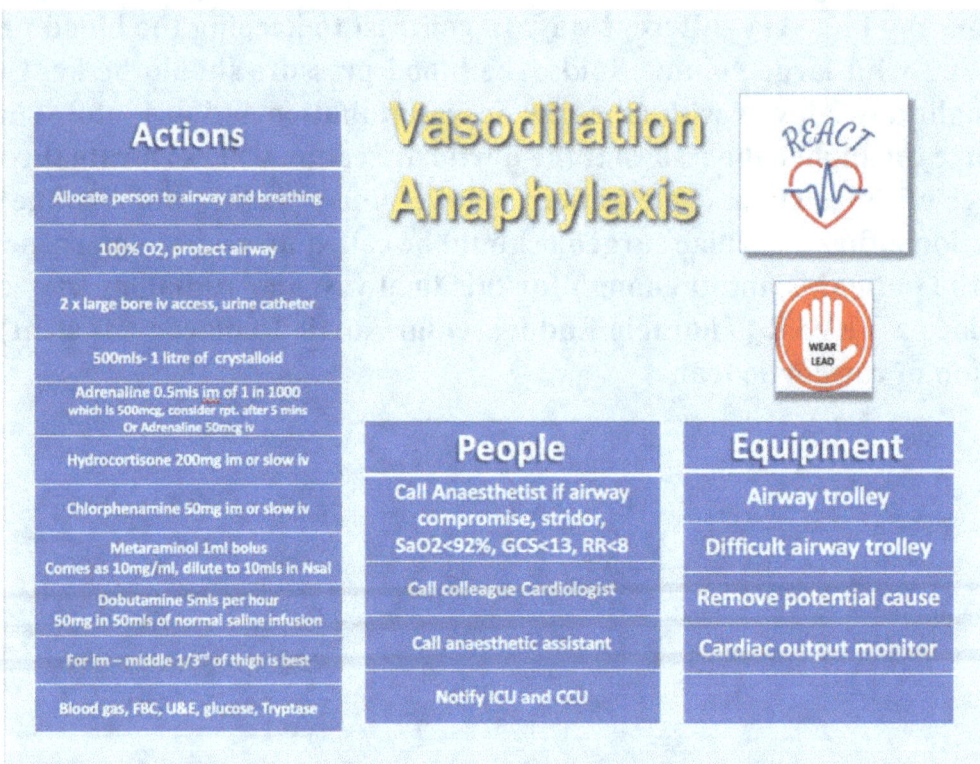

If this emergency is called, then the REACT Team should be formed. A person is allocated to protect the airway and breathing and to give the patient 100% oxygen either through a non-rebreathing mask or a bag valve mask. The flipchart lists a range of medications depending on the severity of the situation. Certainly 500mls of colloid should be given first , and then if there is a significant anaphylactic reaction then 0.5mls of Adrenaline intramuscularly must be given. The alternative would be to administer 1ml boluses of metaraminol (10mg/ml, diluted in 10mls of normal saline). Then hydrocortisone and chlorphenamine may be given. Bloods should be taken and a Tryptase could be considered to see if anaphylaxis was the diagnosis. We have suggested parameters for calling an anaesthetists. If you hear stridor or if there is a reduced conscious level below a GCS of 13 an anaesthetist should be called. If the oxygen saturations are below 92% on 100% oxygen or the respiratory rate is less than 8 breaths per minute then an anaesthetist should be called and they may need both the airway trolley and the difficult airway trolley, and an experienced assistant or operating department practitioner. Some thought should be given to the cause and this should be removed or disconnected from the patient. If there are no other recent or likely medications then the angiography contrast should be considered as the causative drug.

Pulmonary Oedema or Heart Failure

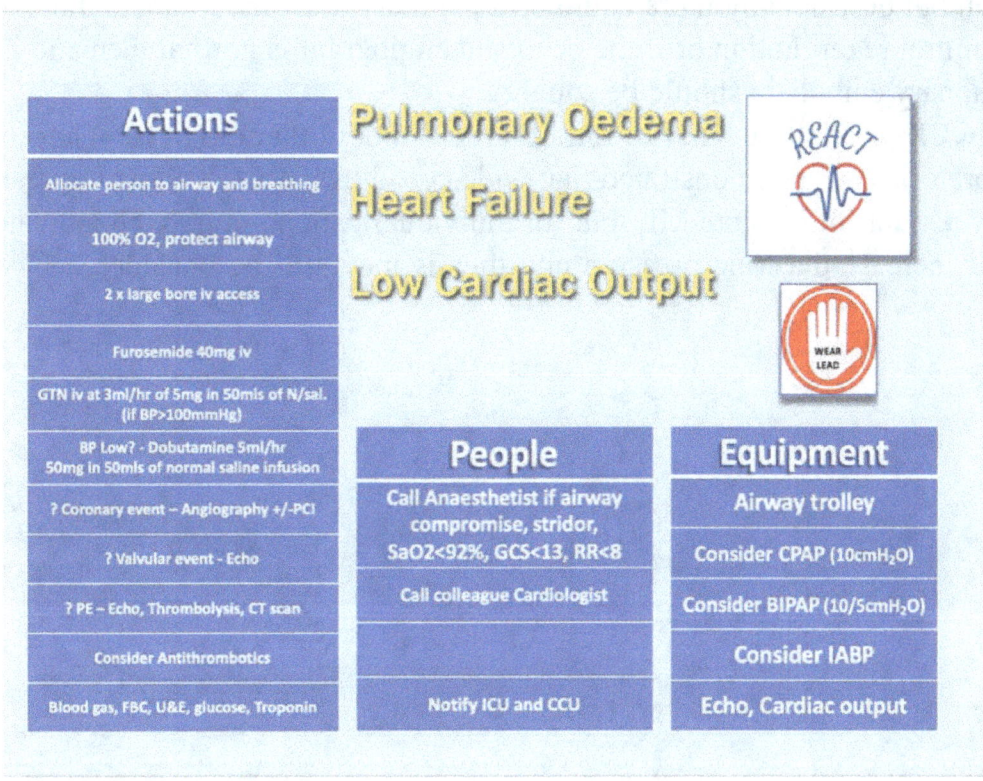

Actions	Pulmonary Oedema / Heart Failure / Low Cardiac Output	
Allocate person to airway and breathing		
100% O2, protect airway		
2 x large bore iv access		
Furosemide 40mg iv		
GTN iv at 3ml/hr of 5mg in 50mls of N/sal. (if BP>100mmHg)		
BP Low? - Dobutamine 5ml/hr 50mg in 50mls of normal saline infusion	**People**	**Equipment**
? Coronary event – Angiography +/-PCI	Call Anaesthetist if airway compromise, stridor, SaO2<92%, GCS<13, RR<8	Airway trolley
? Valvular event - Echo		Consider CPAP (10cmH2O)
? PE – Echo, Thrombolysis, CT scan	Call colleague Cardiologist	Consider BIPAP (10/5cmH2O)
Consider Antithrombotics		Consider IABP
Blood gas, FBC, U&E, glucose, Troponin	Notify ICU and CCU	Echo, Cardiac output

This is not an uncommon emergency in the catheter lab especially with Primary Angioplasty for patients having a myocardial infarction who may come into the catheter lab in fulminant pulmonary oedema and severe heart failure.

If this emergency is called, then the REACT Team should be formed. A person is allocated to protect the airway and breathing and to give the patient 100% oxygen either through a non-re-breathing mask or a bag valve mask. Remember that in pulmonary oedema, the pulmonary venous pressure is raised as the heart cannot keep up with blood coming from the lungs which is the reason for the oedema. Thus CPAP increases the pressure in the alveoli, which can push some of that oedema fluid back into the capillaries and reduce the severity of the pulmonary oedema. Thus obtaining access to CPAP, or even BIPAP is an easy non pharmacological way to treat pulmonary oedema.

We have set parameters for calling an anaesthetist and in addition to respiratory support they may be useful for advice with the administration of inotropes may also be a good reason to call an anaesthetist or intensivist, especially if the attention of the cardiologist is being taken up with emergency revascularisation.

Good iv access is important and multiple iv access is preferable. If the patient has pulmonary oedema with a good blood pressure then iv GTN with furosemide is a good first step. If the blood pressure is low rather than high then vasodilation will not be possible and instead Dobutamine which is a vasodilator but also an inotrope to stimulate the heart may be preferable.

It is important to check with the cardiologist that the diagnosis is secure. If the Angiogram demonstrates severe disease with thrombus then most often this will be secondary to a myocardial infarction but occasionally there could be a papillary muscle rupture and the patient could have severe mitral regurgitation or if the echo and angiogram is normal then another diagnosis such as pulmonary embolism should be sought.

After the SHOCK-II Trial[38], the use of Intra-Aortic Balloom Pumps (IABPs) has diminished in catheter laboratories, as it demonstrated that widespread use of IABPS did not results in better outcomes for patients after acute MI, but for individual patients it may be indicated to reduce afterload and increase diastolic pressure and thus is may still be considered by the REACT Team.

Tachycardia

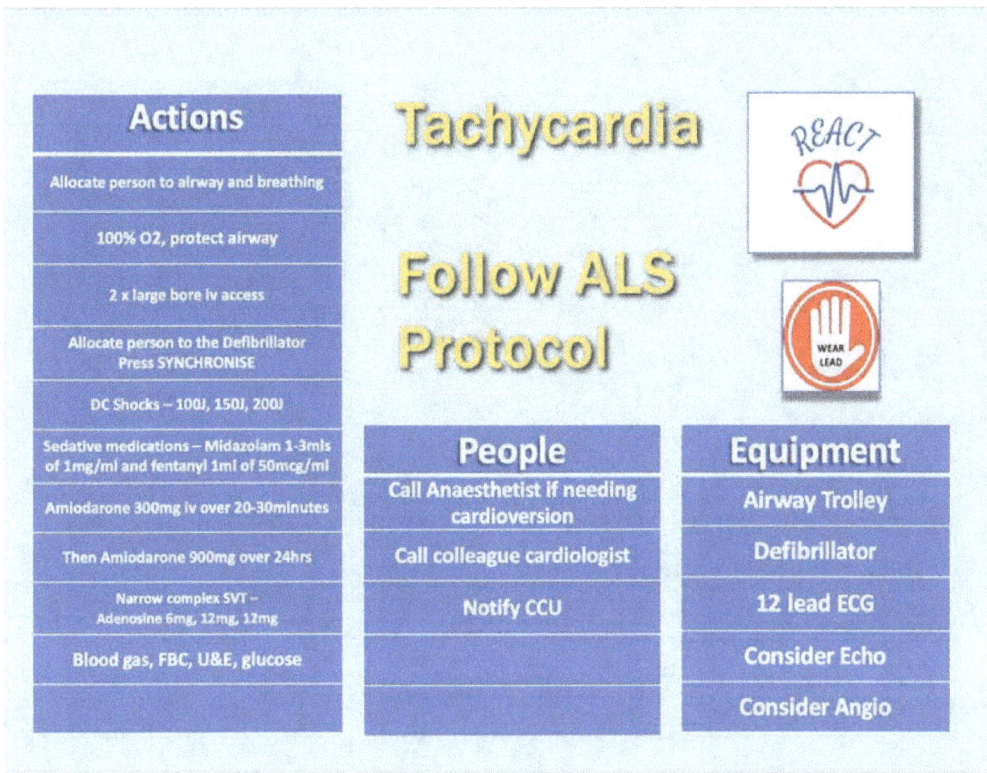

A Tachycardia is often noticed suddenly as patient will often change rhythm quickly or without warning. In a catheter lab it is useful to ask the cardiologist if they thought that they might have caused the arrhythmia as often these are more benign or self-limiting, but nevertheless a REACT Team should be formed.

A person is allocated to protect the airway and breathing and to give the patient 100% oxygen either through a non-rebreathing mask or a bag valve mask. Good oxygenation can sometimes in itself resolve atrial fibrillation or some arrhythmias and so in itself is a treatment for the arrhythmia.

The leader must quickly determine if this is a tachyarrhythmia that requires cardioversion or if it can be treated with medications. This should be communicated clearly to the team and is usually dependent on the blood pressure. A REACT Team member is allocated to stand by the defibrillator and in patients with a pulse it is vital to change its mode to SYNCHRONISE to avoid an R-on-T causing VF after a shock. You should clearly communicate you have done this to the team leader.

If the patient is conscious then sedation is needed for cardioversion. Depending on the level of expertise of the team, it is most usual that an anaesthetist would be required prior to this, as enough sedation is required as to class this as a general anaesthetic. If the patient's blood pressure is very low then it is likely that they will lose consciousness and then cardioversion is immediately performed.

If the rhythm was VT is may indicate myocardial ischaemia and thus angiography should be performed to check for new thrombus and if the patient has been sedated then they may need a higher care environment post procedure than may have been planned.

Bradycardia

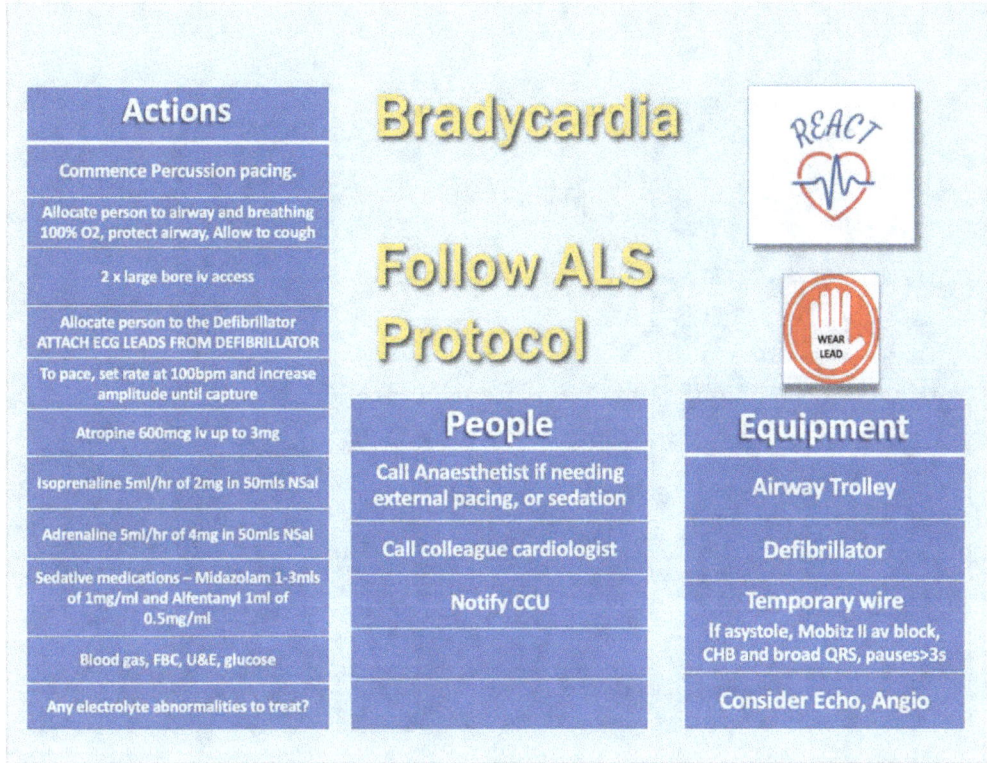

This may occur quickly in response to a vagal stimulation or may happen due to ischemia or an unrelated event. Commonly this may occur in a pacing procedure. The cardiologist may be able to indicate if a wire has cause the emergency or not.

A REACT Team should be formed if simple measures so not resolve the bradycardia. A person should give 100% oxygen via a non-rebreathing mask or a bag valve mask.

Make sure that good iv access is secure. Connect the ECG leads from the defibrillator as a common mistake of external pacing is that the ECG is not connected from the defibrillator and when this machine is changed to pacing mode the trace disappears from the screen and it will not pace, as defibrillators cannot sense and pace at the same time from the pads. Initially if there is a reasonable blood pressure, atropine may be tried up to 3mg, followed by Isoprenaline, and if none of these work then adrenaline is part of the algorithm.

If the blood pressure is very low or these medications have failed then percussion pacing could be tried first, then external pacing followed by a temporary pacing wire. A temporary wire would not require sedation but external pacing would require sedation and therefore an anaesthetist may be required for this.

If there was no obvious cause for the bradycardia then echocardiography and angiography may be advised to seek a diagnosis and consideration of the appropriate location for observation post procedure.

Respiratory Failure

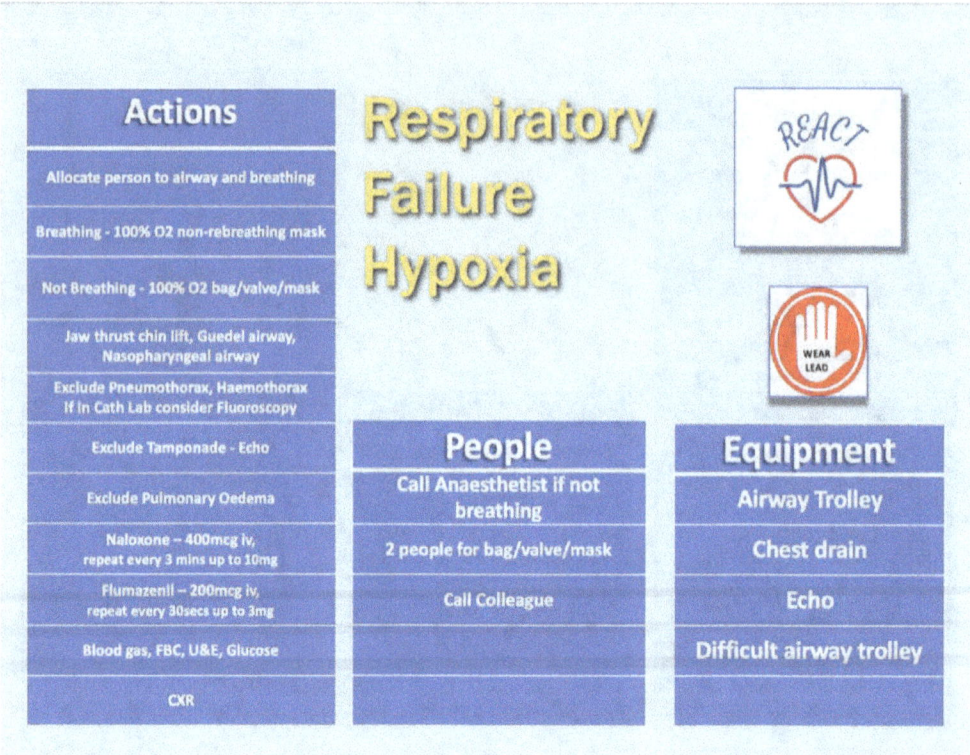

Respiratory failure can be for a variety of causes from Pulmonary Oedema, Pneumothorax, to Bronchospasm or even just oversedation. It is advisable to call for a REACT Team to be formed early and reasonable oxygen saturation should not be used as reassurance as it may be a late sign of respiratory failure especially if oxygen is being given. Abnormal respiratory rate may be an earlier sign or subjective signs of respiratory distress.

1 or even 2 people should be allocated to the airway and breathing and an anaesthetist should be called. Determine whether the patient is breathing or not. If breathing then their own breaths can be supported with 100% oxygen or a bag valve mask held firmly on the face but without trying to force air into the patient. Quickly examine the patient to determine the cause, and specifically look for pulmonary oedema, Haemothorax or pneumothorax or wheeze.

If the patient is not breathing then airway adjuncts are needed to make sure the airway is patent. Similarly seek the cause. In both situations a fluoroscopy can be used to make sure there is not a large pneumothorax.

If no obvious cause is found or if there is pulmonary oedema then an echocardiogram should be performed to see if there is cardiac failure or a tamponade.

In the situation of the patient not breathing if oversedation is suspected, then naloxone or flumazenil will reverse opiates or benzodiazepines.

Vessel Dissection or Perforation

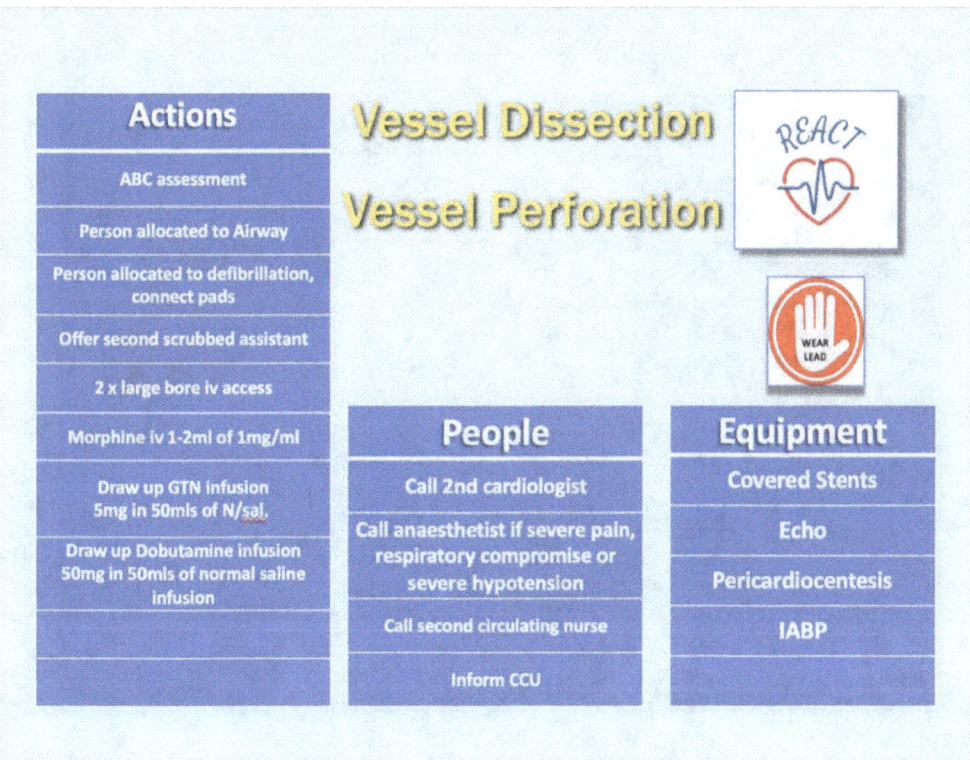

This will most often be called by the cardiologist as often the cardiologist will see this event first. A REACT Team should be formed. A person will go to the head of the patient. If the patient I stable then oxygen may not be required but it would be advisable for the patient to be talked to throughout the procedure so they are aware of the situation. The airway person should be ready to give supplemental oxygen or support the airway in the case of loss of blood pressure.

A person is allocate to the defibrillator and this should be made ready for use if required and a person should be ready to perform CPR if required. A person is allocated to medications. Good iv access should be secured, and that person should be ready to give medications such as morphine, GTN or even dobutamine as necessary.

However one of the most important roles is that of resources. The cardiologist should have an additional scrubbed assistant, and an additional non scrubbed assistant as it is likely that equipment will be required rapidly such as a range of covered stents, occlusion balloons or even pericardiocentesis. In these stressful times, if someone leaves the room or looks for one item then a second person should be available in case the cardiologist needs further equipment rapidly.

Thus additional staff from other cath labs , including scrub staff, runners and also it is adviseable to have another cardiologist to support your cardiologist in this stressful situation.

Pacing Perforation

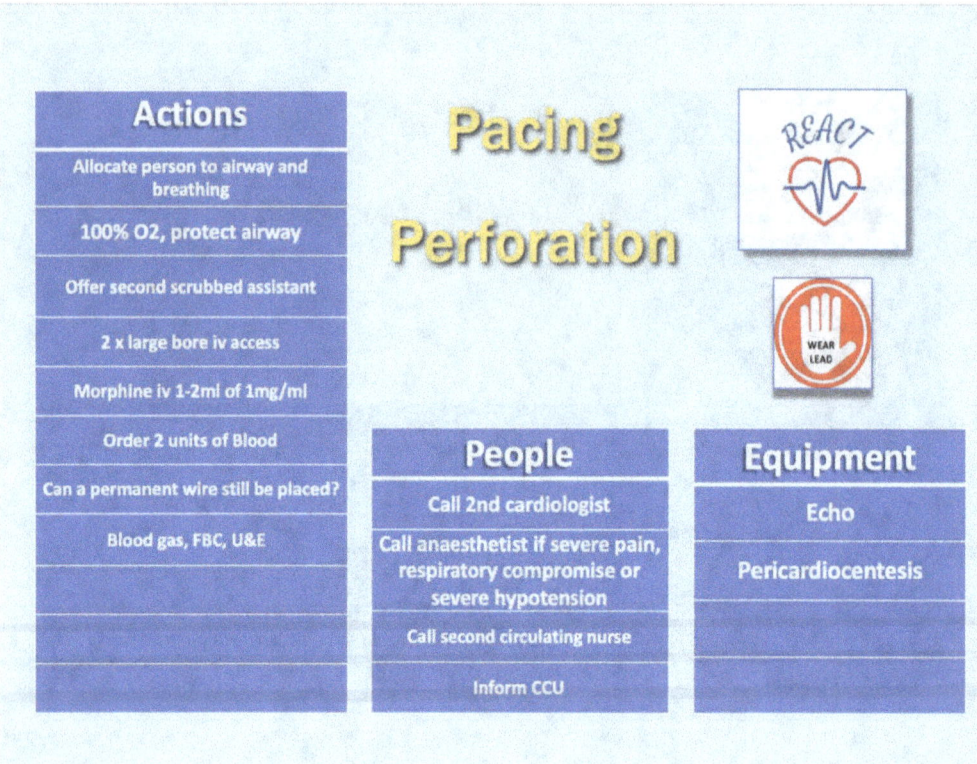

This complication will often be called by the cardiologist who may realise that this has occurred. Alternatively there will be symptoms of either hypovolaemia or more commonly there will be symptoms of tamponade, with hypotension, tachycardia with a cold and clammy patient who may also become breathless. The REACT Team should be formed.

A person will be allocated to the airway and be ready to give supplemental oxygen or support the airway and breathing if the blood pressure drop significantly so that the patient loses consciousness.

A person will be allocated to the defibrillator and be ready to perform CPR but hopefully this will not be required and a person will be allocated to ensure good vascular access and have medications ready such as morphine, or fluids, and potentially inotropes if tamponade has occurred.

But here again the most important roles will be the resource coordination. Additional staff should be called. An additional scrubbed nurse, an additional runner and a colleague cardiologist are vital to ensure that pericardiocentesis may be performed with echocardiography available. Most typically a pericardiocentesis, and relief of the tamponade and removal of the cause and resuscitation of the patient will resolve the situation, but in addition surgical support may occasionally be required if bleeding continues.

If the perforation is controlled then the patient will need a higher observation environment for post procedural observation.

TAVI Annulus Rupture

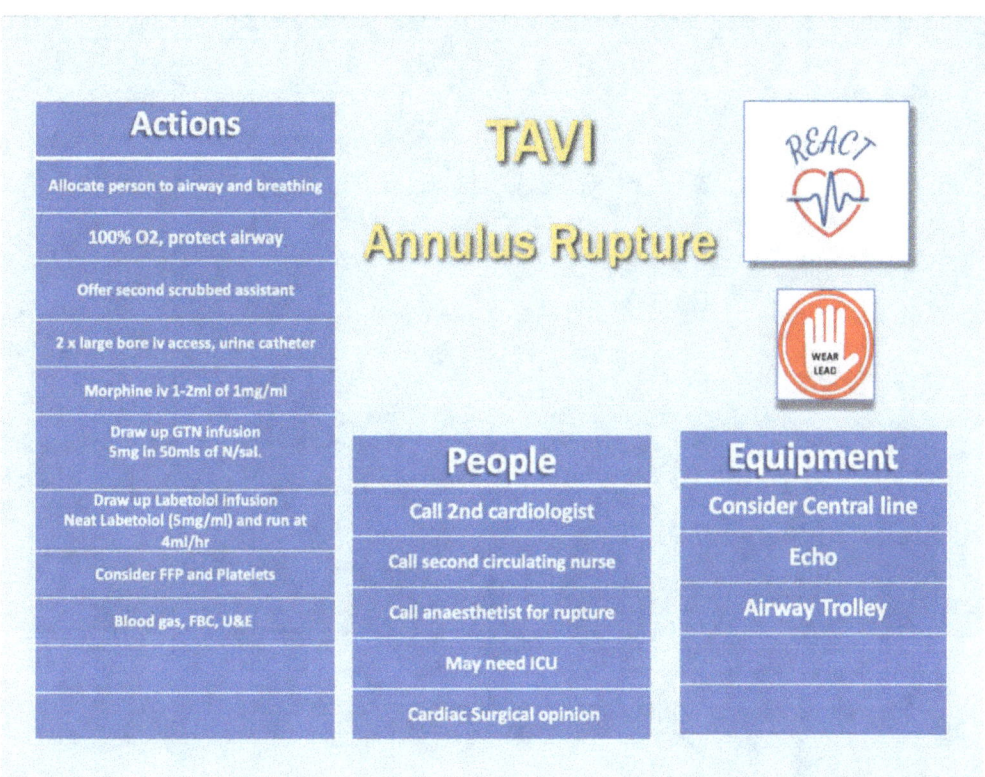

This is a very specialist emergency in the TAVI theatres, and requires a particular protocol for optimal outcome. If the Balloon dilatation of the calcified aortic annulus when the valve is expanded causes an annulus rupture, this is a particular type of aortic dissection directly caused by the balloon expansion. Blood will enter the aortic adventitia, it may occlude the left or right coronary ostium and potentially could cause free wall rupture of the aorta, and tamponade.

The cardiologist will most often identify this complication. Often the patient is having a TAVI as they are high risk for cardiac surgery, but the optimal curative option would be emergency aortic root replacement if the patient was thought to be fit enough for this operation. However most often the patient will not be suitable for emergency surgery. Thus the optimal alternative approach is controlled hypotension, with a general anaesthetic.

A REACT Team should be formed. A person will be allocated to airway and the patient should be pre-oxygenated and talked to and informed of the situation. Preparation should be made for an anaesthetist to intubate and ventilate the patient. A person will be allocated to defibrillator and CPR but hopefully they will not be required. The person allocated to drugs and vascular access will be required to prepare drugs for a general anaesthetic, drugs for maintaining hypotension and adequate vascular access. A central line will be required in this patient at some stage. A second person may have to be allocated to help them. The resource coordinator will also be required to prepare for general anaesthesia and hypotension and transfer to an intensive care unit. An additional scrub nurse and circulating nurse and an additional cardiologist will be very useful also.

Cerebrovascular Accident

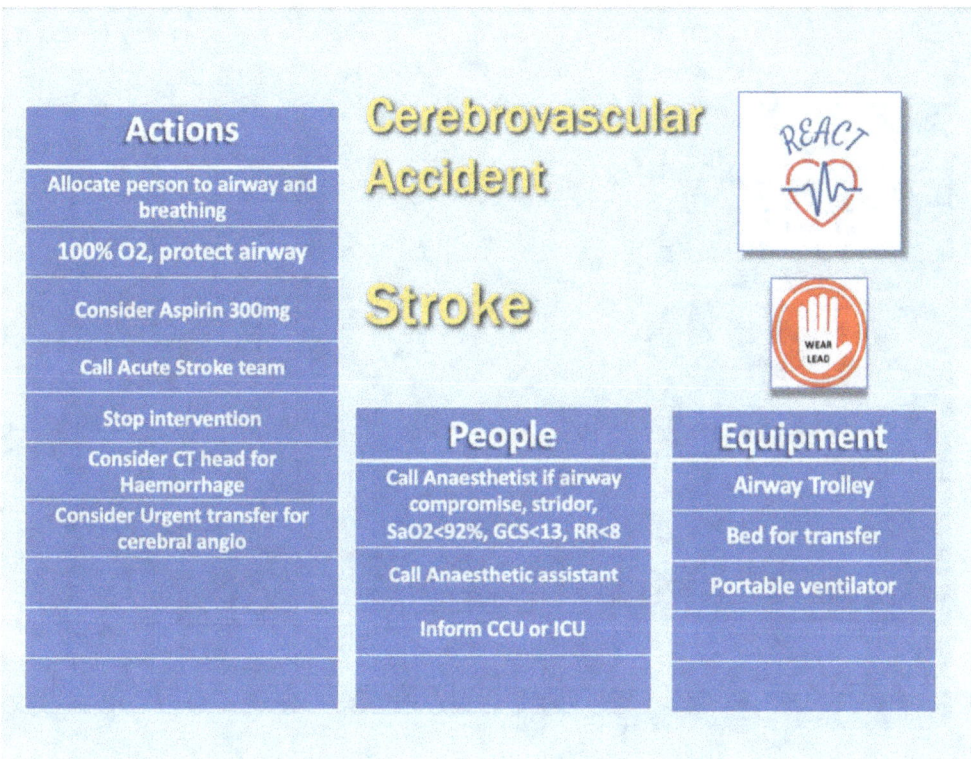

This is a very different complication to the above complications which are mainly complications that cause hypotension or hypoxia. A CVA may manifest itself in many ways. The classic presentation would be dysarthria, dysphasia, hemiplegia, or visual disturbance with or without a headache. But this may not occur as the classical presentation and the patient may suddenly become agitated or confused. The patient may become hypoxic and reduce their respiratory rate, or lose consciousness. If there are any atypical signs or suspicion of a CVA then the REACT Team should be formed.

A person will be allocated to the airway so that the patient is well oxygenated and their breathing is supported if necessary. There will be a person allocated to defibrillation and CPR but often this will not be necessary and thus they could also support the airway team and the patient. The person allocated to drugs and vascular access should investigate the medications that the patient has already had on the communication board and could give aspirin if they have not already had antiplatelets.

We have parameters for calling an anaesthetist and the team leader and the resource coordinator have the opportunity to investigate immediate thrombolysis or cerebral angiography for CVA. This requires a great deal of coordination from multiple teams and the patient will require consultation with neurology, urgent CT scanning and potentially treatment by neurology or neuroradiology. Each department should be aware of their local protocols for immediate stroke treatment.

Bronchospasm

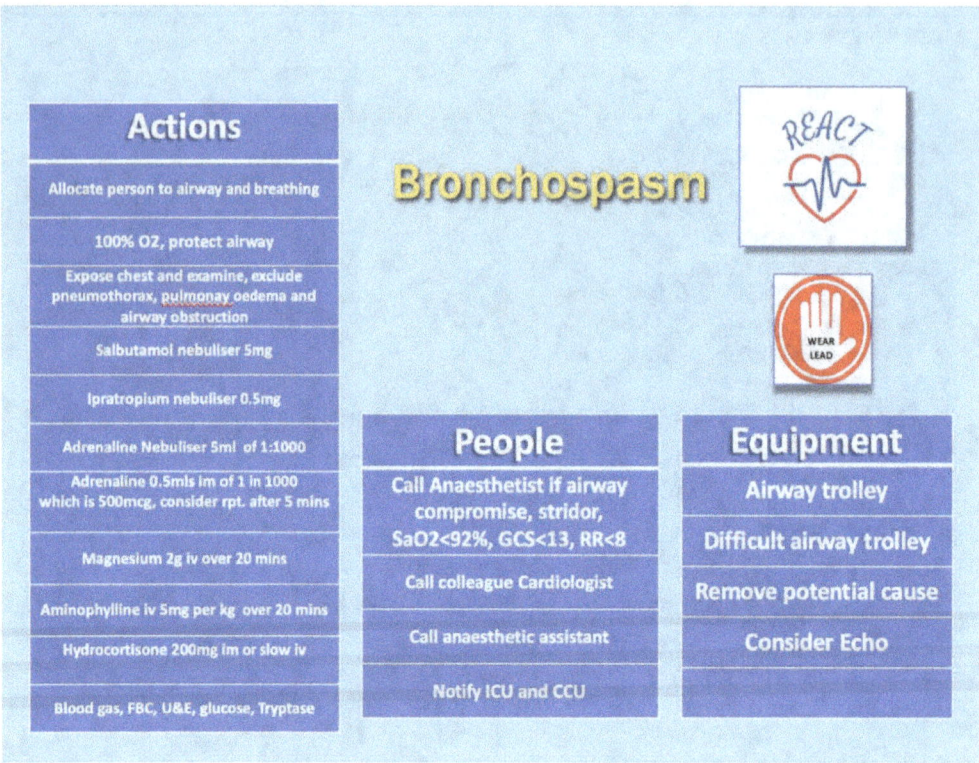

If you hear widespread expiratory wheeze and have hypoxia then bronchospasm may be diagnosed. One or two people should be allocated to the airway and breathing and 100% oxygen applied. Make sure that you and your colleagues are happy with the diagnosis and that there is not an alternative diagnosis such as a pneumothorax (Can take a fluoroscopy image to look at this in addition to clinical signs), pulmonary oedema from heart failure or airway obstruction. We have given here the full algorithm for medications recommended in bronchospasm as each exact dose and the order of administration is not easy to recall in an Emergency. Nebulisers would be the first step, Salbutamol followed by Ipratropium and remember that Adrenaline can be nebulised also. Adrenaline can be given im in the same way that anaphylaxis is treated and Magnesium, Aminophylline and hydrocortisone should also be considered for severe cases.

There will be a low threshold for anaesthetic assessment and help and it may be advisable to check with your anaesthetists if they are happy with the criteria above . If this is agreed then it is simpler to call them in these situations as it has been agreed in advance.

Make sure that both the airway and the difficult airway trolley are available in case of deterioration.

The Joint British Society Guidelines on management of cardiac arrest in the cardiac catheter laboratory

Joint British Societies' guideline on management of cardiac arrest in the cardiac catheter laboratory

Joel Dunning ,[1] Andrew Archbold ,[2] Joseph Paul de Bono,[3] Liz Butterfield,[4] Nick Curzen ,[5] Charles D Deakin,[6] Ellie Gudde,[7,8] Thomas R Keeble,[7,8] Alan Keys,[9] Mike Lewis,[10] Niall O'Keeffe,[11] Jaydeep Sarma,[12] Martin Stout,[13] Paul Swindell,[14] Simon Ray [12]

For numbered affiliations see end of article.

Correspondence to
Professor Simon Ray, Cardiology, Manchester University NHS Foundation Trust, Manchester, Greater Manchester, UK; simon.ray@nhs.net

ABSTRACT

More than 300 000 procedures are performed in cardiac catheter laboratories in the UK each year. The variety and complexity of percutaneous cardiovascular procedures have both increased substantially since the early days of invasive cardiology, when it was largely focused on elective coronary angiography and single chamber (right ventricular) permanent pacemaker implantation. Modern-day invasive cardiology encompasses primary percutaneous coronary intervention, cardiac resynchronisation therapy, complex arrhythmia ablation and structural heart interventions. These procedures all carry the risk of cardiac arrest.

We have developed evidence-based guidelines for the management of cardiac arrest in adult patients in the catheter laboratory. The guidelines include recommendations which were developed by collaboration between nine professional and patient societies that are involved in promoting high-quality care for patients with cardiovascular conditions. We present a set of protocols which use the skills of the whole catheter laboratory team and which are aimed at achieving the best possible outcomes for patients who suffer a cardiac arrest in this setting. We identified six roles and developed a treatment algorithm which should be adopted during cardiac arrest in the catheter laboratory. We recommend that all catheter laboratory staff undergo regular training for these emergency situations which they will inevitably face.

INTRODUCTION

More than 300 000 procedures are performed in cardiac catheter laboratories in the UK each year. The variety and complexity of procedures undertaken in the cardiac catheter laboratory have increased substantially over the last 30 years. Invasive cardiology has grown from a largely diagnostic specialty focused on elective coronary angiography to one that treats a wide spectrum of cardiovascular problems through many different types of interventional procedures, often in urgent or emergency situations. The majority of myocardial revascularisation procedures, for example, are now performed by percutaneous coronary intervention (PCI), and over a quarter of these are undertaken in the setting of acute ST elevation myocardial infarction. Pacemaker implantations have evolved from mostly right ventricular procedures to treat bradycardias to encompass biventricular pacing to deliver cardiac resynchronisation therapy for patients with left ventricular dysfunction and/or implantable cardioverter defibrillators (ICDs) for patients at risk of ventricular arrhythmia. Complex arrhythmia ablation procedures have become more common as their indications and success rates have increased. Recent years have seen a large increase in structural heart interventions driven by transcatheter aortic valve implantation (TAVI) to treat aortic stenosis, adding a further level of complexity to procedures undertaken in the catheter laboratory. Percutaneous interventions on the mitral valve are increasing in number while the tricuspid valve and heart failure syndromes are targets for interventional technology development. Not only have procedures become increasingly complex, they are often undertaken in patients who are elderly and comorbid, with limited cardiorespiratory reserve.

Invasive procedures undertaken in the catheter laboratory all carry the risk of complications which lead directly or indirectly to cardiac arrest. Careful assessment of the risks and benefits of the procedure is required for each patient. In many cases, the risk of cardiac arrest is low. In others, such as primary PCI, the risk is appreciable. The incidence of cardiac arrest during PCI is approximately 1.5%.[1 2] The chance of successful resuscitation is higher than in other in-hospital cardiac arrest situations,[3] especially for elective procedures. The catheter laboratory benefits from the presence of an expert team which is present at the time of cardiac arrest, the reason for the cardiac arrest may be known, and it may be reversible through an intervention in the catheter laboratory. Other specialists are usually readily available to assist, if required. Nevertheless, there is variation between catheter laboratories, for example, whether they are based in a cardiac surgical centre or in a district general hospital and in the number of practitioners and the roles which they undertake in the catheter laboratory. Furthermore, the intervention to achieve restoration of spontaneous circulation (ROSC), such as PCI, may take some time to perform. Rescuers who are used to 10–15 min cardiac arrest scenarios may need to become familiar with prolonged cardiac arrest scenarios which involve mechanical cardiopulmonary resuscitation (CPR), the administration of drug infusions, consideration of every aspect of the patient's physiology, and treatment akin to

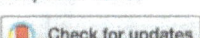
To cite: Dunning J, Archbold A, de Bono JP, et al. Heart Epub ahead of print: [please include Day Month Year]. doi:10.1136/heartjnl-2021-320588

that of a critically ill patient on an intensive care unit (ICU). In undertaking invasive procedures in the catheter laboratory, our expectation should be for successful resuscitation after a cardiac arrest. In aiming to achieve the best possible outcomes, a consistent approach to the arrested patient in the catheter laboratory is needed. For this reason, we have developed evidence-based guidelines for the management of cardiac arrest in the catheter laboratory.

SCOPE AND METHODS

This guideline covers adult patients undergoing any invasive procedure in the catheter laboratory, including coronary angiography, PCI, structural heart interventions including TAVI and mitral valve procedures, pacemaker and ICD implantation, arrhythmia ablation, atrial appendage occlusion, and pacing system extraction. We did not consider patients who suffer a cardiac arrest and are then brought to the catheter laboratory as these patients have recently been considered in a position paper by the European Society of Cardiology (ESC).[4]

The guideline was developed by a collaboration between nine stakeholder organisations: the British Cardiovascular Society (BCS), the British Cardiovascular Intervention Society (BCIS), the British Heart Rhythm Society (BHRS), the British Association for Nursing in Cardiovascular Care, the British Society of Echocardiography, the Association for Cardiothoracic Anaesthesia and Critical Care, the Cardiovascular Care Partnership UK, the Society for Cardiothoracic Surgery in Great Britain and Ireland, and the Resuscitation Council UK.

These guidelines were developed in accordance with The Resuscitation Council UK 2021 guidelines development process.[5] We used the ESC 2018 practice guidelines recommendations for grading the strength of recommendations and for assessing the levels of evidence in support of them.[6] It should be acknowledged that the literature surrounding cardiac arrest comprises mostly of papers which reported the findings of studies after either in-hospital or out-of-hospital cardiac arrest rather than after cardiac arrest in the catheter laboratory and that their findings were extrapolated to the catheter laboratory environment.

We undertook a comprehensive review of the literature and a Delphi expert consensus process in order to identify all of the situations in the catheter laboratory that potentially lead to cardiac arrest and to provide team-based solutions to their management. We propose these guidelines as the standard of care in this specialist area.

The International Liaison Committee on Resuscitation

According to international guidelines, resuscitation is governed by The International Liaison Committee on Resuscitation (ILCOR) which is a collaborative of seven world resuscitation councils which was founded in 1992. The full range of all recommendations in the area of resuscitation is reviewed and updated and a document of the 'best evidence' in resuscitation is created. The seven resuscitation councils then take this evidence and generate guidelines adapted to the needs of their own healthcare systems.

The American Heart Association guidelines

The 2015 American Heart Association (AHA) guidelines contain a two-page section entitled 'Cardiac Arrest During Percutaneous Coronary Intervention', although this was omitted from its 2020 guideline.[7] In 2015 the AHA concentrated mainly on a discussion on the use of automated CPR devices over manual compressions and the use of extracorporeal CPR (ECPR) devices. It did

not come to any firm conclusion but stated that mechanical CPR devices and ECPR devices have been used as bridges to other interventions such as coronary artery bypass surgery, cardiac transplantation or longer-term mechanical devices. In the text of the guideline it is also noted by the authors that early defibrillation within a minute of cardiac arrest is associated with excellent outcomes. No other special considerations were discussed with regard to the management of cardiac arrest in the catheter laboratory.

The European Resuscitation Council guidelines

The European Resuscitation Council (ERC) published guidance regarding resuscitation in the catheter laboratory in 2021 in its document entitled 'cardiac arrest in special circumstances'.[8] It included a protocol diagram, and there was a strong emphasis on ensuring that catheter laboratory staff are adequately trained in resuscitation technical skills including team training, and specific protocols for the initiation of mechanical CPR, temporary pacing and pericardiocentesis, with the use of on-site emergency drills. The ERC also recommended the availability of resuscitation equipment and the use of checklists. Mechanical CPR was recommended due to the risk to staff from manual CPR during fluoroscopy, and the requirement to continue CPR during PCI.

The Australian and New Zealand guidelines

These guidelines discussed the use of mechanical CPR in cardiac arrest during PCI.[9] They also discussed cough CPR for which they found case reports regarding its use during electrophysiology (EP) procedures. They discussed treatment of cardiac tamponade during cardiac arrest by thoracotomy and pericardiotomy if pericardiocentesis fails with a class B recommendation. They noted that the interventionalist is heavily task burdened and, as such, is seldom in a good position to lead the resuscitation and that there may be tension between the requirement to perform CPR and the ability of the interventionalist to continue with the procedure, thus acknowledging two of the particular challenges faced by the catheter laboratory team during a cardiac arrest.

A NOVEL PROTOCOL FOR THE MANAGEMENT OF PATIENTS WHO SUFFER A CARDIAC ARREST IN THE CATHETER LABORATORY

We have developed a modified resuscitation protocol which is specifically designed for the specialist area of the catheter laboratory. Of note this does not apply to recovery areas but does apply to hybrid laboratories where TAVI or Mitraclip procedures are being undertaken. This protocol could also be used in hybrid laboratories performing thoracoscopic endovascular aortic repair (TEVAR). The full protocol is shown in figure 1 and the rationale for its development is discussed.

How should cardiac arrest be identified, defined and categorised?

In a catheter laboratory a cardiac arrest is identified much more quickly than other in-hospital arrest scenarios. Ventricular fibrillation (VF), pulseless ventricular tachycardia (VT) and asystole may be diagnosed immediately when a continuous intra-arterial blood pressure is displayed, without need for an added pulse check.

It is important to define what constitutes a cardiac arrest in a catheter lab. In contrast to the two pathways in the standard arrest algorithm we have separated the protocol into three pathways: VF or pulseless VT, asystole or extreme bradycardia, and pulseless electrical activity (PEA).

Dunning J, et al. Heart 2022;0:1–18. doi:10.1136/heartjnl-2021-320588

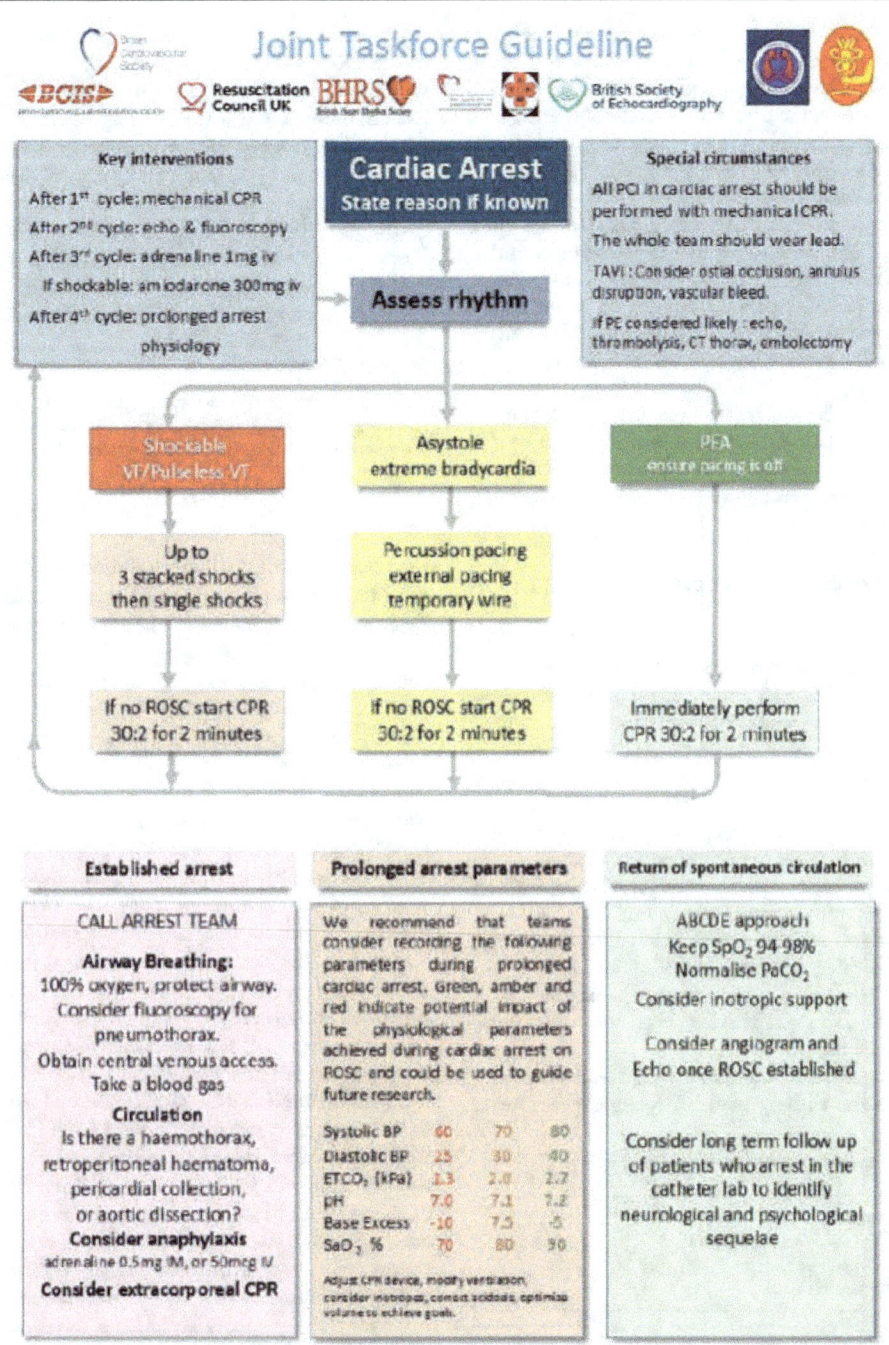

Figure 1 Protocol for resuscitation of patients who suffer a cardiac arrest in the catheter laboratory. BCIS, British Cardiovascular Intervention Society; BHRS, British Heart Rhythm Society; CPR, cardiopulmonary resuscitation; PCI, percutaneous coronary intervention; PE, pulmonary embolus; PEA, pulseless electrical activity; ROSC, restoration of spontaneous circulation; TAVI, transcatheter aortic valve implantation; VF, ventricular fibrillation; VT, ventricular tachycardia.

In VF or pulseless VT, the pulse oximeter and arterial trace will confirm the absence of a cardiac output. A cardiac arrest should be called and the operator should tell the team if they know the reason for the arrest (eg, vessel dissection or occlusion in PCI, occluded left main stem in TAVI or irritation of the ventricle in a pacing procedure for example). VF or VT is occasionally deliberately induced in EP labs and this should not trigger the arrest protocol.

Temporary asystole or extreme bradycardia (<30/min) may occur and can be anticipated during manipulation of ventricular pacing leads or EP catheters. A cardiac arrest should be called when the rhythm disturbance is unexpected and or prolonged. The pulse oximetry and any arterial transduction will show non-pulsatile traces, and percussion pacing, external pacing or temporary wire pacing may be attempted prior to chest compressions.

Many cases of PEA may be diagnosed by the absence of a pulsatile waveform on a continuous intra-arterial blood pressure display. Non-pulsatility or minimal pulsatility of the arterial trace and pulse oximetry in the presence of continuing electrical activity confirms the diagnosis. The operator should call it a cardiac arrest and inform the laboratory team of the likely cause.

Pulseless VT can be mistaken for PEA. A regular rhythm above 140/min should be considered as pulseless VT if the arterial trace and pulse oximetry have minimal or absent pulsation and the patient has lost consciousness. Similarly extreme bradycardia may be mistaken for PEA if the arterial trace is not being transduced. It may be necessary to feel the pulse for 10s or alternatively (and optimally) to perform a rapid echocardiogram to identify a cardiac output.

Occasional patients will deteriorate in the catheter laboratory with support devices in place such as left ventricular assist device (LVAD), extra corporeal membrane oxygenation (ECMO) or Impella (Abiomed), where non-pulsatility does not equate with an absent cardiac output.

Should all members of the resuscitation team wear lead aprons?

All clinicians coming into an arrest in the catheter laboratory should wear lead aprons. Our protocol uses the members of the team present in the catheter laboratory in the initial stages of the arrest and, thus, it is strongly recommended that everyone entering the room should wear lead aprons as it is very likely that the cardiologist may need to perform fluoroscopy in many emergency situations.

We recommend that catheter laboratory team members are regularly trained in basic airway management to ensure a patent airway and good oxygenation for all patients, to ensure that the anaesthetic team have adequate time to put on protective lead before entering the laboratory. We recommend that an individual in the catheter laboratory team is allocated to manage the personnel coming into the arrest. They will be required to assist these personnel to put on lead, and as they do this, they will be able to brief these clinicians as to the arrest situation in the catheter lab.

Catheter laboratories must also ensure that lead aprons in a range of sizes are immediately available for emergency team members.

Recommendation	Class	Level
All clinicians entering a cardiac arrest situation in a catheter laboratory must first put on lead aprons prior to entry. Advance provision should be made for enough lead aprons to be available for this situation.	IIa	C

Should we defibrillate before external chest compressions?

In 2020 ILCOR published a literature review on this subject[10] and it was identified as a priority area for the Basic Life Support Taskforce. They found that in five randomised controlled trials (RCTs)[11 12 13 14 15] there was no difference in outcomes with a specified period of chest compressions (typically 1.5–3 min) before shock delivery compared with shock delivery as soon as possible with interim brief CPR while the defibrillator was readied for use. A meta-analysis of these studies (n=10 600 patients) also found no differences. Only when the arrest time was more than 5 min did any studies show an improvement with CPR before defibrillation.[16 17] The ERC 2021 guidelines[8] do not recommend the routine delivery of a prespecified period of CPR before rhythm analysis and shock delivery, and recommend shock delivery as soon as it can be applied. Deferring chest

compressions until after shock delivery has been recommended in the ERC 2021 guidelines[8] in other highly monitored areas such as after cardiac surgery and these now state: 'If a patient has a monitored and witnessed cardiac arrest (eg, in the catheter laboratory, coronary care unit, or other monitored critical care setting in or out-of-hospital) and a manual defibrillator is rapidly available: Confirm cardiac arrest and shout for help. If the initial rhythm is VF/pVT, give up to three quick successive (stacked) shocks. Rapidly check for a rhythm change and, if appropriate, ROSC after each defibrillation attempt. Start chest compressions and continue CPR for 2 min if the third shock is unsuccessful'.

Recommendation	Class	Level
In ventricular fibrillation (VF) or ventricular tachycardia (VT) without a cardiac output, external chest compressions may be deferred in order to perform up to three stacked shocks immediately.	IIa	A

How many attempts at defibrillation should be performed prior to commencing external chest compressions?

Evidence was sought for the optimal number of attempts at external defibrillation for VF or pulseless VT prior to commencing external chest compressions. This has been subject to a literature review looking at the effectiveness of the numbers of defibrillation attempts in a range of scenarios including ICD insertions, electrophysiological studies, out-of-hospital arrests and animal studies.[18] When the data from all 15 papers are combined, the average success rate of sequential shocks declines from 78% for the first shock to 35% for the second shock and 14% for the third, and any subsequent shock will have less than a 10% chance of success. Thus, the likelihood of successful cardioversion declines dramatically from first to second shock and declines further from second to third shock.

Our guideline seeks to place a mechanical CPR device on the patient early in the pathway and it is important to consider how we modify the protocol to allow this. First, it may be possible to assess the rhythm while the mechanical CPR is ongoing. Our patients often have multi-lead ECG monitoring, and sometimes intracardiac ECG monitoring, and thus where the team leader is satisfied that there has been no change from the shockable rhythm, there is no need to pause the CPR device every 2 min. If the team leader is uncertain then a pause should be performed every 2 min for rhythm assessment. As there is no risk to a rescuer, charging and administration of a shock may be performed while mechanical CPR is ongoing. Finally, if multiple shocks have failed to cardiovert the patient and it is clear that a coronary occlusion is the cause of the arrhythmia, then mechanical CPR should continue uninterrupted until coronary flow is restored.

Recommendations	Class	Level
In ventricular fibrillation (VF) or pulseless ventricular tachycardia (VT), up to three stacked shocks should be given without intervening external chest compressions.	I	B
Thereafter, a single attempt at defibrillation, if required, is performed every 2 min.	I	C
If the arrhythmia is due to an acute coronary artery occlusion, repeat shock administration can be deferred to facilitate percutaneous coronary intervention (PCI) to the occluded artery.	IIa	C
Shocks for known VF/VT should be administered while mechanical cardiopulmonary resuscitation (CPR) is ongoing.	I	C
If the patient is receiving mechanical CPR and it is possible to assess the rhythm while the CPR is ongoing then it may not be necessary to pause the CPR device.	IIa	C

Should we perform pacing in patients who undergo an asystolic arrest in the catheter laboratory prior to external chest compressions?

In an asystolic arrest in a catheter laboratory there is the potential to rapidly restore cardiac output with pacing and, as this is a witnessed arrest, if pacing is performed immediately then potentially there will be an immediate restoration of a spontaneous circulation. Furthermore, in the literature review on the effectiveness of external chest compressions in the early stages of an arrest[19] it was found that there was little evidence to suggest harm from delaying external chest compressions for a few minutes. Periods of asystole are not uncommon in pacing and electrophysiology (EP) laboratories and most cardiologists would use external, percussion or transvenous temporary wire pacing to address this as a routine part of their practice. We recommend that pacing should be attempted prior to the initiation of external chest compressions.

Percussion pacing may initially be attempted (see the section below for further details). For external pacing the pacing pads should be applied, and the amplitude of the pacing quickly increased to regain an output. Only if capture is not obtained with maximum amplitude with the pads well applied should external chest compressions be performed. If the cardiologist suspects that the arrest is due to an extreme bradycardia due to a conduction defect then transvenous pacing can be used if external pacing has been ineffective in achieving ventricular capture.

Recommendations	Class	Level
In a patient who arrests with asystole or extreme bradycardia with a rate of less than 30 bpm, external pacing or percussion pacing should be attempted prior to chest compressions.	IIa	C
If either external or percussion pacing is ineffective and the cardiologist feels that there is a persisting bradycardia as the cause of the arrest a temporary pacing wire should be inserted while chest compressions are performed.	IIa	C

Interventions to address PEA

Our protocol using three categories aims to ensure that the greatest number of patients possible may benefit from either immediate defibrillation or pacing prior to the institution of external cardiac compressions. In patients presenting with PEA efforts should be directed towards identifying the underlying causes and treating them rapidly. There are a number of possibilities to consider that are relevant to the catheter laboratory:

Hypoxia: There is an airway and breathing protocol with a person allocated to address these issues in an arrest.

Hypovolaemia: bleeding. Our recommendation ensures that the four most likely areas for bleeding in the catheter laboratory (haemothorax, retroperitoneal or vascular bleed, aortic dissection and tamponade) are investigated.

Hypo/hyperkalaemia, H^+ ion imbalance and electrolyte abnormalities are addressed by a recommendation to perform an early blood gas.

Hypothermia is unusual in a catheter lab, other than following prolonged out of hospital arrest

Tension pneumothorax may arise during procedures requiring vascular access in the thorax. This is addressed in the airway and breathing protocol and by fluoroscopy.

Tamponade: Where tamponade is a possibility immediate echocardiography should be performed. The clinical sign most suggestive of tamponade in a cardiac arrest is the inability to generate a systolic blood pressure of 70 mm Hg with external cardiac massage.

Toxins: One possible cause of a toxin-related arrest in a catheter laboratory is a drug error. We recommend that any syringe drivers or infusions should be stopped in the arrested patient to address this possibility. Careful consideration should also be given to contrast-induced or antibiotic-induced anaphylaxis. Look for supportive signs such as rash, wheeze or facial swelling. Our protocol recommends epinephrine 0.5 mg intramuscular or otherwise 50 mcg intravenous.

Thrombosis: coronary or pulmonary. In the catheter laboratory this would most commonly relate to acute coronary occlusion, either due to an acute myocardial infarction or a complication of PCI which in both circumstances would be treated by reopening of the vessels by PCI. Pulmonary embolism causing an arrest is far less common. In an arrest situation it can be very difficult to diagnose but is suggested by disproportionate right ventricular distention. If suspected, then thrombolysis or thrombectomy might be considered. This is considered in our protocol.

How deeply should we perform chest compressions?

The universal algorithm recommends compressing the chest to between 5 cm and 6 cm over the lower half of the sternum.[7 8] For those patients with an arterial trace being transduced, we recommend 'titrating' chest compressions to achieve a systolic pressure of 70 mm Hg. This allows more gentle external compressions to be performed, potentially reducing the chance of compression related injury, while still producing effective cerebral perfusion. Furthermore, the inability to generate an acceptable systolic pressure is suggestive of tamponade.

Recommendations	Class	Level
Chest compressions should be performed to a depth of 5–6 cm to the lower half of the sternum.	IIa	C
If the arterial trace is being transduced it is preferable to compress to achieve a systolic pressure of 70 mm Hg.	IIb	C

Should we perform a precordial thump?

The AHA guidelines[20] state that 'The precordial thump may be considered for termination of witnessed monitored unstable ventricular tachyarrhythmias when a defibrillator is not immediately ready for use (Class IIb, level of evidence (LOE) B), but should not delay CPR and shock delivery'. ILCOR produced a worksheet on this subject in 2021.[21] This documents that precordial thump is only effective in 2% of attempts and, in fact, rhythm deterioration is twice as common as successful cardioversion. Thus, our protocol does not recommend a precordial thump. A defibrillator should be immediately at hand in every catheter laboratory, and this is much more likely to successfully cardiovert the patient.

Recommendation	Class	Level
A precordial thump is not recommended for patients who suffer a cardiac arrest in the catheter laboratory due to ventricular fibrillation (VF) or pulseless ventricular tachycardia (VT).	III (no benefit)	C

Is cough CPR an effective alternative to external chest compressions in the catheter laboratory?

The AHA stated in 2010 that 'cough' CPR may be considered in settings such as the cardiac catheterisation laboratory for conscious, supine and monitored patients if the patient can be instructed and coached to cough forcefully every 1–3 s during the initial seconds of an arrhythmic cardiac arrest. It should not delay definitive treatment (Class IIb, LOE C). The AHA made no modifications to this recommendation in 2020.[7]

The longest documented case of a patient maintaining their own spontaneous circulation is 90s and most reports were around 30s, in both VF as well as asystole. These patients seem able to maintain consciousness in a manner similar to the mechanism proposed for external CPR, namely a compression of the pulmonary vascular bed increasing the pressure in the left atrium then ventricle and allowing blood to flow across the aortic valve.[22] There are case reports of its use for short periods of time in the catheter laboratory,[23] including prior to defibrillation[24 25] but the most effective use seems to be in patients with severe bradycardia who are periarrest. ILCOR performed a systematic review in 2021.[21] Their conclusion was as follows: 'We suggest cough CPR may only be considered as a temporising measure in an exceptional circumstance in a witnessed, monitored, in-hospital setting (such as a cardiac catheterisation laboratory) if a non-perfusing rhythm is recognised promptly before loss of consciousness (weak recommendation, very-low-certainty evidence)'.

If a bradycardic or asystolic cardiac arrest is very rapidly identified (while the patient is responsive), then it is reasonable to attempt to coach the patient to cough forcefully every 1–3s if experienced clinicians choose to try this. This should not delay the commencement of the cardiac arrest protocol including the application of pads and defibrillating or pacing if necessary. Staff should be ready to perform CPR if the patient stops following the command to cough, and the arterial trace should be observed to monitor the effectiveness of cough CPR.

Recommendation	Class	Level
Vigorous cough cardiopulmonary resuscitation (CPR) every 1–3s in the catheter laboratory may only be considered as a temporising measure if a non-perfusing rhythm is recognised promptly before loss of consciousness. It is likely to be most useful in bradycardia in order to maintain consciousness until more definitive reversal measures can be instituted.	IIb	C

Percussion (fist) pacing as an alternative to CPR in the catheter laboratory

ILCOR performed a systematic review on this subject in 2021.[21] The total number of cases reported in the literature is around 170 patients and in the largest series of 100 patients, 69 of these maintained consciousness and 90 had percussion pacing as an alternative to CPR.[26]

In a study performed in 1978[27] 19 healthy volunteers and 31 patients with paused pacing had a right heart catheter and the authors found reliable electrical impulses could be reproduced for up to 6 min when the left lower sternum was struck with the clenched fist from about 20–30 cm height, by causing the right ventricular pressure to rise by around 20 mm Hg with this action.

The ILCOR 2021 systematic review states that 'We suggest fist pacing may only be considered as a temporising measure in an exceptional circumstance in a witnessed, monitored, in-hospital setting (such as a cardiac catheterisation laboratory) if a non-perfusing rhythm is recognised promptly before loss of consciousness'.

The catheterisation laboratory is a highly monitored environment where bradycardia and asystole are common. There have been no studies comparing CPR to percussion pacing directly but percussion pacing has been shown to effectively induce cardiac contraction and maintain consciousness in patients immediately identified as having an asystolic arrest. Therefore, with close

monitoring, we recommend that this could be a useful temporising method in the catheterisation laboratory, while preparations are made for external pacing or a temporary wire or the administration of chronotropic medications.

Recommendations	Class	Level
In monitored patients with onset of a non-perfusing rhythm such as asystole or extreme bradycardia (figure 1), percussion (fist) pacing may be deployed as an alternative to external pacing when successful perfusion is confirmed by a continuous arterial tracing, pulse oximetry and ECG.	IIb	C
Percussion pacing should be performed at a rate of 50–70 per minute and the ulnar side of a clenched fist should be used to strike the chest from 20–30 cm above the left lower sternal edge, in order to mechanically increase the right atrial pressure, if measured, by 15–20 mm Hg.	IIb	C

Active pad compression for defibrillation

In atrial fibrillation there are papers including the Ottowa AF Cardioversion protocol[28] and the 2014 AHA guidelines for the management of patients with atrial fibrillation[29] that mention using paddles to provide manual compression over the defibrillator pads as a method of increasing the success of cardioversion. The original citation as evidence in favour of this intervention was by Kerber et al[30] in 1981 looking at 44 cardioversion patients, although, interestingly, the only part of this paper that actually looked at active compression was a subreport of four dogs who were cardioverted with or without active compression.

Sirna et al in 1988 reported a 13% reduction in impedance with active compression when uniphasic defibrillation was being performed in 28 patients[31] and a similar result was found by Ramirez et al in 2016 with 11 participants where they concluded that 8 kg of pressure could reduce the impedance by about 10%.[32]

Thus, there is limited evidence from animal studies and case series, as well as a trial of cardioversion in atrial fibrillation, that active compression of the defibrillation pads using disconnected defibrillation paddles reduces intrathoracic impedance and improves shock efficacy. In the absence of any studies in ventricular arrhythmias in humans the routine use of active compression during defibrillation is not recommended. However, the use of disconnected defibrillation paddles to apply external compression to defibrillation pads may be considered in patients with arrhythmias refractory to cardioversion particularly where there is a risk of high intrathoracic impedance.

Recommendations	Class	Level
Active pad compression is not routinely recommended for defibrillation and the standard method of defibrillation should be via pads either in an anterior-lateral position, an anterior-posterior position or apex-posterior position.	III (lack of benefit)	C
In situations when initial attempts at cardioversion have failed, an expert clinician who feels that increased impedance may be a factor, such as in high body mass index (BMI), may elect to try active pad compression if paddles are also available to provide the compression.	IIb	C

Does epinephrine improve outcomes in resuscitation in the catheter laboratory?

ILCOR in 2015 reviewed the literature with regard to epinephrine including a large RCT by Olasveengen et al[33] where ambulances were randomised to Group 1: CPR and defibrillation with iv cannulation and usual resuscitation medications versus Group 2: CPR and defibrillation alone. This RCT showed reduced survival to hospital discharge in Group 1 and this was felt to be due to the ineffectiveness of the drugs and also the delay in CPR in order to cannulate and administer the drugs. This paper, and a more recent meta-analysis[34] (demonstrating no benefit of epinephrine in cardiac arrest) led ILCOR to write: 'despite the widespread use of epinephrine during resuscitation, and several studies involving vasopressin, there is no placebo controlled study that shows that the routine use of any vasopressor at any stage during human cardiac arrest increases survival to hospital discharge. Current evidence is insufficient to support or refute the routine use of any particular drug or sequence of drugs. Despite the lack of human data, the use of epinephrine is still recommended, based largely on animal data'.

The PARAMEDIC-2 Study[35] randomised 8014 patients in an arrest situation across five ambulance services in the UK to receive either 1 mg of epinephrine every 3–5 min, or identical syringes containing 0.9% saline. The mean time for the ambulance to arrive was 6.6 min and the mean time to trial drug administration was 13 min after arrival. There was a large increase in the number of patients who had return of spontaneous circulation in the epinephrine arm (36% vs 11%), as well as the number who were transferred to hospital (50% vs 30%). The primary outcome measure was survival at 30 days and this was 3.2% in the epinephrine group and 2.4% in the placebo group which was significant, but the number of survivors with severe neurological impairment was 31% in the epinephrine group versus 18% in the control group, and thus the trial was negative in terms of survival with favourable neurological outcome (2.2% vs 1.9%). The triallists concluded that epinephrine significantly improved the chance of achieving the return of spontaneous circulation and the survival of the patient to hospital admission but that it led only to a greater proportion surviving with severe neurological disability.

In the light of this important study, we suggest that the current recommendations of giving epinephrine every 3–5 min at a dose of 1 mg is supported on the basis that it is unlikely to harm the patient and may be beneficial. We recommend that intravenous epinephrine (1 mg) is given after the third cycle. It may be acceptable to administer smaller doses of epinephrine if a senior clinician feels that there may be reactive hypertension on ROSC.

The guideline group also discussed the question of the administration of epinephrine in cases of a non-shockable rhythm. Current recommendations from the ERC are to give epinephrine at a dose of 1 mg as soon as possible but they do caveat this by saying that 'exceptions may exist where a clear reversible cause can be rapidly addressed'. In PEA and asystole in the catheter laboratory there are reversible causes that should be addressed, and for this reason the group concluded that we should recommend administering epinephrine at the same time as in a shockable rhythm to allow time for reversible causes to be addressed.

Recommendations	Class	Level
We recommend that for patients who arrest in a catheter laboratory the benefits of epinephrine which are mainly based on out-of-hospital arrest randomised controlled trials (RCTs) may also apply in terms of an increased return of spontaneous circulation.	I	A
We recommend that for patients who arrest with ventricular fibrillation (VF) or pulseless ventricular tachycardia (VT) intravenous epinephrine 1 mg is given after the third shock cycle.	I	A

Table 1 Physiological parameters of interest.

Physiological parameters of interest

The following parameters are suggested to encourage data collection and stimulate research in a cardiac arrest management. It should be noted that they are not known markers of improved clinical outcome.

Parameter of interest	Parameter targets		
Systolic blood pressure (mm Hg)	60	70	80
Diastolic blood pressure (mm Hg)	25	30	40
Central venous pressure (mm Hg)	5	10	20
Coronary perfusion pressure (mm Hg)	10	15	20
End-tidal CO_2 (mm Hg)	10	15	20
End-tidal CO_2 (kPa)	1.3	2	2.7
PH	7.0	7.1	7.2
Base excess (mmol/l)	−10	−7.5	−5
Oxygen saturation (%)	70	80	90
Cerebral oximetry (Near infrared spectroscopy) (%)	25	30	40

Green, amber and red indicate potential impact of the physiological parameters achieved during cardiac arrest on restoration of spontaneous circulation (ROSC) and could be used to guide future research. Clinical decisions regarding cessation of resuscitation should not be based only on these parameters.

Recommendations	Class	Level
We recommend that for patients who arrest with a non-shockable rhythm intravenous epinephrine 1 mg is given after the third cycle of cardiopulmonary resuscitation (CPR) rather than immediately to allow time for reversible causes of cardiac arrest to be addressed	IIa	C

Waveform capnography in cardiac arrest

We recommend that waveform capnography is used for patients in established cardiac arrest. Not only does this prove that the airway is patent, and that there is reasonable air entry to allow the exchange of CO_2, but more importantly the level of exhaled CO_2 correlates with the cardiac output. Capnography can be used as a prognostic guide to the likely result of prolonged resuscitation. An end-tidal CO_2 more than 20 mm Hg (2.7 kPa) is a good prognostic indicator whereas an end-tidal CO_2 of less than 10 mm Hg (1.3 kPa) indicates a poor prognosis and may be used to indicate that further treatment is likely to be futile or that modifications are required to the CPR to improve this figure.

Goal-directed management during prolonged cardiac arrest in the catheter laboratory

A number of physiological parameters are associated with higher rates of ROSC. This has led to the hypothesis that higher rates of ROSC and better clinical outcomes might be achieved by goal-directed resuscitation techniques. This may be particularly relevant to the management of cardiac arrest in the catheter laboratory where resuscitation attempts may be prolonged and invasive monitoring is routine.[36 37 38] Physiological parameters of interest based on our literature review on this topic are listed in table 1. This concept was investigated in a series of 10 patients who underwent mechanical CPR and PCI to treat prolonged cardiac arrest in the catheter laboratory.[39] The average time of mechanical CPR was 43 min. Systolic blood pressures above 70 mm Hg and diastolic blood pressures above 40 mm Hg were targeted. A pigtail catheter was inserted into the right atrium via the femoral vein at the interventionists discretion to monitor CVP and to administer vasoactive drugs. The investigators aimed to keep the CVP below 25 mm Hg. If this was not achieved, echocardiography was performed to exclude cardiac tamponade, the mechanical CPR device was repositioned, and inotropes or vasoconstrictors were initiated. End-tidal CO_2 was measured following insertion of an endotracheal tube or a supraglottic airway with a target of >15 mm Hg (>2 kPa). The SpO_2 was kept above 80%, and arterial blood gas measurement was used to guide 'normo' ventilation. Cerebral oximetry was also monitored. Vasoconstrictor infusions were used in favour of epinephrine boluses. For patients in VF, attention was directed towards opening the acutely occluded coronary artery in favour of repeated attempts at defibrillation. The protocol was simulated in training prior to its institution. Early experience identified difficulties measuring all of the parameters every 2 min during ongoing cardiac arrest. When the parameters were measured successfully, they regularly identified patients whose vital parameters were suboptimal.

In the AHA 'get with the guidelines registry' of 3023 monitored cardiac arrests and 6064 unmonitored in-hospital cardiac arrests, those who had a monitored arrest had a significantly better chance of survival based mostly on blood pressure and end-tidal CO_2 monitoring.[40] The AHA recommended keeping the end-tidal CO_2 above 20 mm Hg and the diastolic blood pressure above 25 mm Hg in their consensus statement on improving resuscitation outcomes.[41]

A group in Greece wrote a discussion document proposing the 'PERSEUS' protocol in 2019 aimed at prolonged physiological monitoring of patients in cardiac arrest.[42] They proposed mechanical CPR, and ventilating the patient with positive end expiratory pressure (PEEP) of zero, respiratory rate of 10 per min, tidal volume 6 mL//kg, 100% oxygen, inspiration:expiration ratio 1:2. In a previous observational study they had found higher airway pressure was associated with better outcomes, with a pressure of 40–45 mm Hg giving optimal outcome. They discuss the pitfalls of using end-tidal CO_2 to estimate cardiac output and discuss how positive pressure ventilation may be used to augment cardiac output during chest compressions. They suggested placing a CVP line with the aim being to keep the CVP below 25 mm Hg and advocated that if the CVP was low, a straight leg raise should be performed to assess volume status and then fluid be given as indicated. They suggested using optimal positioning of the mechanical CPR device and epinephrine infusions to keep the diastolic blood pressure above 40 mm Hg and that severe acidosis be treated immediately to prevent vasodilation and decreased central perfusion pressure.

Among over 1500 patients with out-of-hospital cardiac arrest in whom a venous blood gas was measured, adverse results were associated with a lower rate of survival. In particular, patients without ROSC had a mean pH of 7.11, pCO_2 of 9.7 kPa, base excess of −7 mmol/L, potassium of 4.5 mmol/L and a lactate of 7 mmol/L. Low pH, high pCO_2 and high plasma potassium concentration were predictors of poor outcome.[43]

A meta-analysis of goal-directed resuscitation identified mainly animal studies but did conclude that goal-directed CPR may be superior to standard CPR, especially when end-tidal CO_2 and blood pressure management were targeted.[44] It is important to emphasise that a low end-tidal CO_2 may reflect inadequate ventilation rather than low cardiac output, especially when a supraglottic airway is used, because of the higher airway pressures required during chest compressions and steps should be taken in these cases to place an endotracheal tube as soon as it is safe to do so.

Monitoring of the CVP allows an estimate of coronary perfusion pressure by subtracting the diastolic arterial pressure from the CVP. Ideally it should be kept above 20 mm Hg.

The catheter laboratory is a unique environment in which physiological parameters can be accurately monitored during circulatory arrest. These parameters can be used to assess the effect of interventions such as the adjustment of cardiac massage technique, intravenous administration of vasoactive medications, correction of acidosis, electrolytes, and volume status, and less conventional treatments such as head-up CPR, while prolonged revascularisation attempts are ongoing or preparation is made for ECPR. Whether or not goal-directed resuscitation improves clinical outcomes, or even increases rates of ROSC, is not yet clear so firm recommendations for setting physiological parameter targets during cardiac arrest cannot be made. Nevertheless, we recommend that teams consider recording physiological parameters during prolonged cardiac arrest (table 1). Green, amber and red indicate the potential impact of the physiological parameters achieved during cardiac arrest on ROSC and could be used to guide future research. Clinical decisions regarding cessation of resuscitation should not be based only on these parameters.

Recommendation	Class	Level
We recommend that physiological parameters are recorded at regular intervals during cardiac arrest in the catheter laboratory once mechanical cardiopulmonary resuscitation (CPR) has been instituted.	IIb	C

Is amiodarone of use in a VF arrest in the catheter laboratory?

We sought evidence as to whether amiodarone or lidocaine may be useful for VF/pulseless VT. There is good evidence in support of Amiodarone in four large randomised trials,[45–48] each demonstrating an improvement of the chance of successful cardioversion of about 10%. It must be noted that these studies are all in the out-of-hospital setting and thus there is less certainty that the results might be equivalent in the in-hospital setting or indeed in a catheter laboratory.

Amiodarone should be given as a bolus injection of 300 mg. A further dose of 150 mg may be given for recurrent or refractory VF/VT followed by an infusion of 900 mg over 24 hours. Lidocaine 1 mg/kg may be used as an alternative and may have a similar efficacy.[49] There is less robust evidence regarding alternatives such as procainamide.

Recommendation	Class	Level
After three failed cycles of defibrillation for ventricular fibrillation (VF) or pulseless ventricular tachycardia (VT) without a cardiac output, a bolus of 300 mg of intravenous amiodarone should be administered.	I	A

The use of echocardiography during cardiac arrest

Echocardiography can help to identify the cause for the arrest and should be performed rapidly as an integral part of the resuscitation. It is important to exclude tamponade early in the resuscitative process and also to repeat the echo in a prolonged arrest if the effectiveness of CPR diminishes abruptly as this may indicate tamponade secondary to external cardiac massage or delayed onset of tamponade. Echocardiography has also been shown to reduce the time taken for pulse checks[50] by enabling visualisation of the presence or absence of organised contractions.

In patients who already have a transoesophageal echo (TOE) probe in place this has advantages compared with transthoracic echocardiography[51] in that it does not require interruptions of CPR, can be performed continuously with better images, can be used to identify ROSC quickly, to look for dissection of the ascending aorta and, if required, can aid placement of pacing wires or the initiation of ECPR. It is also better at monitoring the effectiveness of prolonged mechanical CPR. In addition, there may be clinicians experienced in its use available in the

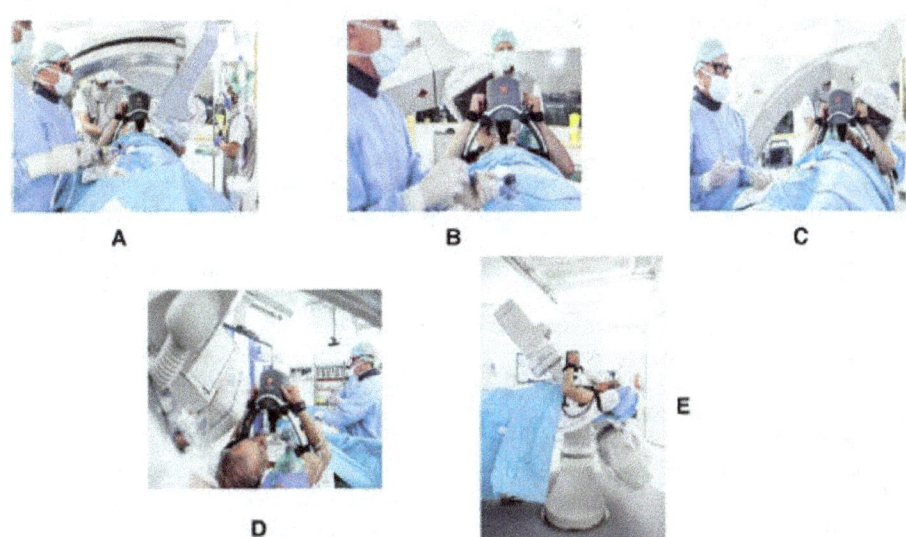

Figure 2 Fluoroscopic projections possible with the automatic external cardiac massage device in place. (A) Right posterior oblique; (B) Left anterior oblique; (C) Right anterior oblique; (D) Straight cranial; (E) Straight caudal (with permission from Stryker Corporation).

Recommendations	Class	Level
We recommend that teams undergo regular group training to ensure that the transfer from manual CPR to automated CPR is conducted in less than 15 s.	I	C

ECPR in the catheter laboratory

The AHA and the ERC both recommend the use of ECMO to provide ECPR. The AHA state that 'rapid initiation of eCPR or cardiopulmonary bypass is associated with good patient outcomes in patients with haemodynamic collapse and cardiac arrest in the catheter laboratory and also the use of eCPR is feasible and associated with good outcomes when used as a bridge to coronary artery bypass grafting' (AHA Class IIb, LOE C). The ERC are more equivocal, stating that very low quality evidence suggests that the use of extracorporeal life support can be considered as a rescue strategy if the infrastructure is available, and this should probably be preferred to the use of intra-aortic balloon pump (IABP) in such situations. The First RCT in this area called the ARREST Trial was stopped early due to the highly significant effects in favour of ECMO in out of hospital cardiac arrest (OHCA). Thirty patients were randomised and there were six survivors in the ECMO group compared with only one in the standard care group.[71] Furthermore, there are many case series reporting the efficacy of extracorporeal cardiopulmonary bypass[72-80] in the context of catheter laboratory based cardiac arrests. Bagai et al reported in 2011 on the use of extracorporeal cardiopulmonary bypass in 39 patients in a range of situations including cardiac arrest and cardiogenic shock in the catheter laboratory. The survival to discharge was 71%.[76] Van den Brink in 2018[80] reported the use of extracorporeal cardiopulmonary bypass in 12 patients of whom 11 were in cardiac arrest with a survival to discharge of 67% and a 1-year survival of 42%. Nine had out-of-hospital arrest and a further two had in-hospital arrest.

The Extracorporeal Life Support Organisation has published a position paper in 2018, advocating ECMO in arrests of longer than 15 min of duration, but centres offering ECMO are required to be looking after at least 30 patients a year and therefore will generally be located only in transplantation centres.[81]

Recommendation	Class	Level
It is recommended that units investigate the use of ECMO as a further means of supporting patients who do not recover after cardiac arrest in the catheter laboratory and have local protocols and training in place for its effective use if it is available.	IIa	B

IABP insertion in the arrest situation

The evidence for the insertion of an IABP in an arrest situation was reviewed. Of note the AHA have also reviewed this evidence and concluded that while IABP counterpulsation increases coronary perfusion, decreases myocardial oxygen demand and improves haemodynamics in cardiogenic shock states, it is not associated with improved patient survival. They state that the role of IABP in patients who have a cardiac arrest in the catheterisation laboratory is not known.

The IABP-SHOCK II Trial which randomised nearly 600 patients who were in shock from an acute myocardial infarction did not find an improvement in the 30-day survival after the intervention.[82] This landmark study followed 13 RCTs together with meta-analyses and a Cochrane systematic review which were all unable to detect a significant improvement in 30-day survival although other small improvements were sometimes reported.[83-90] It must be noted that although these studies were in patients with an acute myocardial infarction (rather than patients in cardiac arrest in a catheter laboratory) the IABP-SHOCK Trial has led to a significant reduction in the use of IABP in cardiogenic shock in catheter laboratories.

A further small RCT looking at IABP versus control in patients who suffered a cardiac arrest with an acute coronary syndrome also found no benefit.[91]

There are few studies looking at the insertion of IABPs in the arrest situation.[92 93] Without a spontaneous circulation to trigger the IABP, counterpulsation would be unlikely to be successful. Thus, it is concluded that there is no indication to place an IABP acutely in the cardiac arrest period in the catheter laboratory.

Recommendation	Class	Level
The insertion of an intra-aortic balloon pump (IABP) during an arrest in the catheter laboratory or routinely in the acute postcardiac arrest period is not recommended.	III (lack of benefit)	A

Is an Impella pump useful in an arrest?

The ERC in 2015 stated in their section on cardiac arrest in the catheter laboratory that 'There is no evidence to recommend circulatory support with the Impella pump only during cardiac arrest' and in 2021 they changed this slightly to say that they may provide circulatory support while performing rescue procedures but require further evaluation. They provided a single reference to support this[94] which was a case series of eight patients who had an Impella device in an arrest, of whom four survived to hospital discharge. We identified a further paper documenting use in 7 patients in arrest, although only 1 survived,[95] and a multicentre study across four countries[96] of 35 patients having Impella insertion while in cardiac arrest with a 45% survival.

There have been case series and cohort studies of the use of the Impella in cardiogenic shock in adults and children[97] and in high-risk PCI cases[98–100] and there is an interesting ongoing RCT currently recruiting that aims to randomise 360 patients with shock post-myocardial infarction (MI) to standard therapy or Impella that will report in the coming years.[101]

The 2021 joint ERC and European Society of Intensive Care medicine guidelines for postresuscitation care state that 'the evidence about which type of mechanical device is superior appears inconclusive and thus their use should be decided on a case-by case basis'.[95]

Recommendation	Class	Level
The use of an Impella is not routinely recommended in cardiac arrest in the catheter laboratory	III (lack of benefit)	C

The identification and treatment of pericardial tamponade

Sethi et al reported the findings of the US National Inpatient Sample database from 2009 to 2013 which covers around 90% of all patients in the USA. They document 64 000 pericardiocentesis procedures and 57% of these were in unstable patients, 17% were in PCI cases, 13% in EP procedures and 14% in structural heart procedures. Thus, pericardiocentesis is performed in all types of catheter laboratory interventions.[102] As this was a database study they were unable to comment on the procedural success rate, although the inpatient mortality in the database overall was around one in four.

Tsang et al documented a 21-year experience with a thousand pericardiocentesis procedures at the Mayo clinic, including many patients with perforation in the catheter laboratory. They report a 97% procedural success for this procedure in all settings with only a 2% major complication rate. They also reported that they saw a significant increase in the rate that clinicians left a drain in situ during the period of the study from 25% to 75%.[103]

Cho et al confirmed these findings in a report of nearly 300 echocardiographically guided pericardiocentesis procedures, with approximately 40 during PCI. They reported a 99% procedural success with a 1% complication rate.[104]

A UK observational study of 270 329 PCI procedures in the context of acute coronary syndromes describes 1013 coronary perforations (0.37%).[41] Importantly, the adjusted ORs for all clinical outcomes were adversely affected by coronary perforation. The conclusion was 'Coronary perforation is an infrequent event during ACS-PCI but is closely associated with adverse clinical outcomes'.

The ESC position statement on the urgent management of cardiac tamponade[105] gives a class I indication for pericardiocentesis for tamponade, preferring echocardiographic guidance where possible although fluoroscopic guidance is an acceptable alternative. If unsuccessful, surgical drainage is recommended. Of note these guidelines are mainly for non-iatrogenic causes of the tamponade

It is extremely important that all catheter laboratories have immediate access to an echo machine in order to be able to confirm or exclude tamponade in an emergency. All cardiologists who perform interventional procedures should be trained in pericardiocentesis techniques, and all catheter labs should have a dedicated and easily accessible pericardiocentesis kit, which the team are familiar with. The emergency procedures for pericardiocentesis should be familiar to all catheter laboratory staff. The pericardiocentesis/perforation kit should be stored together and include drainage equipment, coils and covered stents. There should be an agreed unit protocol as to the method of distal embolisation technique as a wide variety of options are available.

In all cases of pericardial collection, repeat TTE should be performed within 2 hours of return to the ward and often again within the following few hours. This is particularly important in the case of distal wire perforations and any case in which a perforation has apparently sealed spontaneously.

Recommendations	Class	Level
Pericardiocentesis should be performed for all patients with pericardial tamponade and where possible this should be with echocardiographic or fluoroscopic guidance. Surgical drainage and repair should be performed if percutaneous drainage is not successful in relieving the tamponade.	I	B
An echocardiography machine should be immediately available in all catheter laboratories in case of patient deterioration or arrest.	I	C
We recommend that a repeat echocardiogram is performed to reassess the pericardial space after drain insertion to monitor for recurrence of a haemopericardium.	IIa	C

Treatment of pericardial tamponade if pericardiocentesis fails

A BCIS analysis from 2006 to 2013 of the complete UK PCI database reported a 0.3% perforation rate with PCI.[106] This comprised of 1762 patients of whom 14% developed tamponade (246 pts) and 3% required emergency surgery (52 patients). Thus, there are roughly 250 coronary perforations per year with around 35 associated episodes of tamponade and seven patients per year in the UK who require emergency surgery after coronary perforation.

This number is likely to have increased since 2013. Furthermore, this database does not include pacing procedures, EP or structural heart procedures. Thirty-seven per cent of coronary perforations occurred in a unit without surgical cover (589 coronary perforations in units without on-site surgical cover compared with 997 in units with cover). Coronary perforations can be classified using the Ellis Classification both in the arrest and the non-arrest situation according to the significance of the defect created in the artery.[107]

With regard to the perforation of cardiac chambers from non-PCI interventions, the National Cardiovascular Data Registry in the USA[108] documented 625 cardiac perforations in a 5-year period, which was one perforation for every 700 implantations of an ICD. The BHRS has provided detailed guidance in their 2016 document entitled 'Standards for Interventional Electrophysiology and catheter ablation in adults'.[109]

We recommend that for coronary perforations consideration be given to heparin and antiplatelet reversal, a decision that must be balanced against the risk of producing stent thrombosis. An activated clotting time could be used to guide this decision.

We recommend there should be on-site availability and experience with covered stents, embolisation coils and the ability to perform distal embolisation. There should be an agreed unit protocol as to the method of distal embolisation technique as a wide variety of options are available.

For perforation of cardiac chambers we also recommend consideration of reversal of heparin, calling for senior colleague assistance, where relevant withdrawal of the lead or wire from the perforation and echocardiographic monitoring for a tamponade.

Recommendations	Class	Level
For coronary perforations, consideration should be given to reversal of anticoagulants, antiplatelet medications and glycoprotein IIb/IIIA inhibitors and an activated clotting time (ACT) should be performed.	IIb	C
There should be on-site availability and experience with covered stents, embolisation coils and the ability to perform distal embolisation. There should be an agreed unit protocol as to the method of distal embolisation technique as a wide variety of options are available.	IIa	C
For all cardiac perforations, even if the patient seems stable, a decision must be taken as to whether cardiac surgical colleagues should be consulted. The threshold for surgical discussion should be low. Failure to stop the underlying cause for the tamponade should mandate emergency consultation.	IIa	C

Surgical support

There should be access to emergency cardiothoracic surgery for all patients who have suffered a tamponade in the catheter laboratory. In units without cardiac surgical cover, an agreed written protocol must be in place in order to ensure that timely relief of a tamponade is possible. The time taken for a patient to sternotomy should be of a similar order to that possible with on-site surgical facilities where a surgical team is not on stand-by.

Options to achieve this may include rapid transfer to the cardiothoracic centre with surgeons ready to receive the patient, or using experienced on-site surgeons trained in emergency thoracotomy to commence relief of a tamponade while a cardiac surgeon travels to the local centre. We recommend that these protocols be documented and tested regularly to ensure equitable availability of potentially life-saving interventions in both centres with and without on-site cardiac surgical cover.

We furthermore recommend the notification of the on-call surgical team for all coronary perforations that cannot be sealed via percutaneous techniques, and all cardiac chamber perforations requiring a pericardiocentesis drain, even if they seem stable, so that the most appropriate management strategy can be agreed.

Recommendation	Class	Level
In units without cardiac surgical cover, an agreed written protocol must be in place in order to ensure that timely surgical relief of a tamponade is possible. The time taken for a patient to sternotomy should be of a similar order to that possible with on-site surgical facilities where a surgical team is not on stand-by.	IIa	C

The management of pulmonary embolus

We identified papers relevant to the management of either confirmed or suspected pulmonary embolus (PE) in cardiac arrest. In addition, the ESC have guidance on the treatment of PE[110] and the AHA and ERC both give recommendations in this area.

It may be difficult to determine PE as the cause of the cardiac arrest although in-hospital arrest teams have been able to identify PE up to 85% of the time.[111] Teams may identify factors precipitating the cardiac arrest before the actual arrest which may include a high-risk history such as malignancy, previous PEs or recent surgery, they may identify symptoms such as dyspnoea, tachycardia and chest pain, and there maybe signs on ECG or a distended right ventricle on echocardiography prior to the arrest.

Once the arrest has occurred, the arrest rhythm is more commonly PEA (63%) versus only 5% in VF.[112] Echocardiography during the cardiac arrest may identify a distended right ventricle with a flattened interventricular septum in cases of PE large enough to precipitate arrest,[113] although right ventricular dilatation in arrest should be interpreted with caution.[114]

In terms of the treatment of the PE in the cardiac arrest Li et al published a meta-analysis in 2006[115] of eight papers that demonstrated that thrombolytics administered during CPR did improve survival, although inevitably there was also an increase in bleeding complications. In an RCT of 1000 patients with out-of-hospital arrests randomised to thrombolytic therapy, no improvement in survival was seen but the percentage of patients who actually had PE may have been low in this study.[116]

The ERC recommend the use of fibrinolytics for patients suspected of arresting secondary to a massive pulmonary embolus.[8] They also recommend that CPR should then continue for 60–90 min and that a mechanical compression device may therefore be required for this. In addition, if there is return of spontaneous circulation then particular attention should be paid to identification of bleeding complications thereafter and in centres where this is available ECPR could be considered.[117–122]

The AHA gives a class IIb indication for echocardiography during cardiac arrest stating that 'if a qualified sonographer is present and use of ultrasound does not interfere with the standard cardiac arrest treatment protocol, then ultrasound may be considered as an adjunct to standard patient evaluation'. The AHA recommend thrombolysis with a class IIb strength of recommendation in addition to systemic anticoagulation. The AHA also mention the possibility of percutaneous mechanical thrombectomy although many units would not have access to this as it requires specialist equipment. One case series reported a successful outcome of percutaneous mechanical thrombectomy during CPR in six out of seven patients.

We also discussed whether in an arrest where PE is suspected in the catheter laboratory pulmonary angiography should be performed, but technically this was felt to be difficult to perform.[123]

Recommendation	Class	Level
In confirmed or suspected acute massive pulmonary embolus in the catheter laboratory, we recommend thrombolysis and systemic anticoagulation. Cardiopulmonary resuscitation must then continue for 60–90 min. Echocardiography may assist in making this diagnosis.	IIb	B

Dunning J, et al. Heart 2022;0:1–18. doi:10.1136/heartjnl-2021-320588

Return of spontaneous circulation

Once there has been a return of spontaneous circulation a full airway, breathing, circulation examination should be performed. Angiography and echocardiography should be considered where appropriate. If the patient has not neurologically recovered sufficiently or their gas exchange is unfavourable it is often safer to intubate and ventilate. Appropriate vascular access with a central line and an arterial line will allow cardiac monitoring and vasoactive drug use as necessary. It is important that such patients are treated in an intensive care area environment if ventilated and at least a high care area otherwise. If there has been a prolonged period of arrest then targeted temperature management has been extensively investigated especially in out-of-hospital arrests[124] and may help a patient who has had a prolonged arrest. However there have been no in-hospital studies to demonstrate benefit and the target temperature has not been established and therefore routine early cooling is not recommended.

Perhaps more importantly the possible longer-term effects of arresting in the catheter laboratory should be considered. If the patient makes a good physical recovery, they should be fully counselled as to the events that occurred in the arrest and consideration of additional or prolonged follow-up should be given to make sure that they suffer no neurological or psychological sequelae. The ERC and the European Society of Intensive Care Medicine have written detailed guidance in 2021 for post-resuscitation care which addresses many of these issues[125] and in addition to this there is excellent patient support at the website www.suddencardiacarrest.org.

THE OPTIMAL CONFIGURATION FOR THE CARDIAC ARREST TEAM

In order to carry out emergency protocols efficiently, whether they be in an arrest situation or with a deteriorating patient, it is vital for all team members to know their roles and responsibilities. There may be a wide variety of staff numbers and skill mixes available in the catheter laboratory area depending on the size of the institution and also the time of day or night. Therefore, there will clearly also have to be some flexibility and also additional roles that might be allocated, but we propose these six key roles to allow a structure for people to work towards (Figure 3). In addition, it is optimal that the staff members will know in advance the role that they would be expected to take in an emergency, and that this could be documented on a communication board at the start of a shift.

The operator

While the cardiologist takes the lead in the catheter lab, the main aim of our protocols is to free this person up of responsibility for resuscitation in the cardiac arrest or the emergency situation. The cardiologist should stay scrubbed at the side of the patient. They are often the person to see the emergency first, and thus must declare this early to the team but thereafter an emergency team leader should be allocated.

The cardiologist is best placed to perform the specialist interventions that may resolve the situation. They should concentrate on this aspect of the pathway and coordinate with the other staff addressing resuscitation via the team leader.

Role 1: The emergency leader

We recommend that someone other than the operating cardiologist organise the team to achieve the best outcome for the patient. We do not mandate who this person should be in terms of their discipline or qualifications, and in fact we are of the opinion that everyone who works in a catheter laboratory should be trained to be able to carry out each of the six key roles, although often in the day there might be another senior cardiologist who will be available to perform this role.

The role is to coordinate the protocols highlighted above as the leader of the group addressing all the components of the arrest response. The leader is encouraged to have the protocol to hand on a flip chart or on a poster.

The emergency leader must make sure personnel are allocated to all required roles and will also allocate tasks to additional people, outside of the six key roles

Role 2: Airway and breathing

If there is any acute emergency and especially in an arrest, the scrubbed personnel will be dealing with the circulation, so

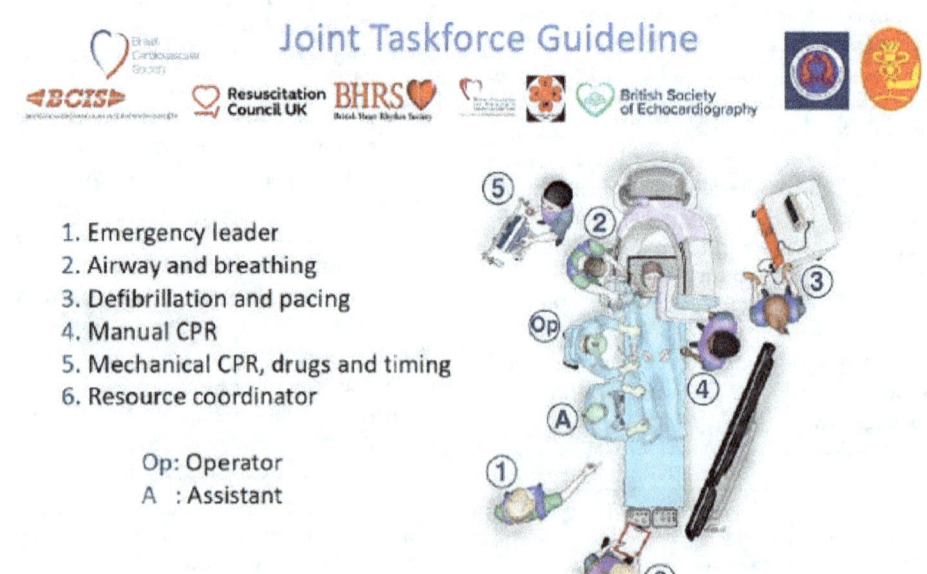

Joint Taskforce Guideline

1. Emergency leader
2. Airway and breathing
3. Defibrillation and pacing
4. Manual CPR
5. Mechanical CPR, drugs and timing
6. Resource coordinator

Op: Operator
A : Assistant

Figure 3   The six key roles. BCIS, British Cardiovascular Intervention Society; BHRS, British Heart Rhythm Society; CPR, cardiopulmonary resuscitation.

another member of staff should go straight to the head of the patient to take responsibility for airway and ventilation. For a person who is not breathing they must immediately get a bag/valve/mask at 100% oxygen and place this on the patient's face and attempt to ventilate the patient. If they are successful, then the chest will rise on both sides, and water vapour may be seen in the mask. If they are unsuccessful then an airway obstruction issue must be considered. Attempt airway manoeuvres—jaw thrust, chin lift, Guedel airway and perhaps ask another person to help with squeezing the bag so you can use two hands to form a good seal around the patient's nose and mouth. We do not recommend that staff who are not fully trained in the technique attempt intubation. In most instances simple airway manoeuvres and airway adjuncts will suffice. A supraglottic airway is a recommended alternative to intubation. Emergency call-out for anaesthetic support is mandatory in this situation.

Once air entry is established in an arrest you must coordinate 30:2 with the person performing massage or the automated CPR device. Your role also requires you to feel the trachea to see if it is central or displaced and then ask everyone to stop massage and bag forcefully while listening bilaterally to see if you can hear a difference in breath sounds.

It is mandatory to perform these assessments in every critically ill catheter laboratory patient if you do not know the cause of their deterioration, and you must communicate that you have done this to the team leader. It is not always easy to, but if you are getting air entry from bagging but it is more difficult than you would expect, if the trachea is not central and if you bag vigorously but cannot hear breath sounds on one side then a pneumothorax or haemothorax should be suspected and this must be communicated to the team leader. We also recommend that fluoroscopy is performed for every arrested patient without an obvious cause for the arrest.

If a tension pneumothorax is suspected, for example, oxygen saturations dropping and the patient complaining of being short of breath before becoming periarrest or arresting during a pacing procedure, then needle thoracocentesis should be performed followed by a drain or a thoracostomy.

Role 3: Defibrillation and pacing

We recommend that a single person is always allocated to this role and stays beside the defibrillator at all times, even if the rhythm is not shockable. The person fulfilling role 3 should place pads on the patient wherever it is most convenient. Often they will be draped and therefore access will be limited but this will have been practised in simulation so should not be an issue. Anterior-lateral position, an anterior-posterior position or apex-posterior positions are all acceptable.

Where the rhythm is shockable we recommend immediate three-stacked shocks. Once the first shock has been delivered, external cardiac massage should not be recommenced, but the rhythm assessed while the defibrillator is being charged for the next shock. If there is no ROSC and the rhythm remains shockable, up to two further shocks should be delivered in rapid succession. The defibrillator operator is responsible for communicating to the team when the defibrillator is charging and before each shock.

If the third shock fails then further shocks may be given at 2 min intervals as determined by the resuscitation leader and the operating cardiologist. Most defibrillators when turned on, activate a timer, so the defibrillator operator is often the best person to time the CPR cycles.

Role 3 is also important in the two other rhythm disturbances. In asystole or extreme bradycardia without a pulse, external pacing may rapidly resolve the situation. We recommend that percussion pacing is attempted while pads are placed on the patient, and it is also important that defibrillators cannot pace and sense from the same pads and thus it is mandatory that ECG leads are placed on the patient and connected to the defibrillator prior to attempting external pacing. We recommend that external cardiac massage is withheld until the pacing is attempted. When the pacing is activated on the defibrillator it usually defaults to the minimum amplitude, and therefore this will have to be increased to achieve capture. If capture is not achieved at maximum amplitude then it is unlikely to work unless the pads are poorly placed and the attempt can cease. If it is felt likely that the asystole or extreme bradycardia could be resolved with pacing, and both percussion and external pacing were unsuccessful then the final option would be a temporary wire to be placed in an arrest situation by the cardiologist.

Defibrillation is not required in PEA arrest but the defibrillator operator should ensure that underlying VF or asystole is not mistaken for PEA in patients with either a temporary or permanent pacemaker in place. We are aware of three cases when this occurred and although rare, if there is a temporary wire with pacing this can be paused to check, or if there is a permanent pacemaker then a relatively narrow QRS complex with a regular rate should raise this suspicion.

Role 4: Manual chest compressions

One person should be allocated to perform CPR. If there are very limited numbers of people in the room at night then either the cardiologist or the scrub nurse could do this but it is an important role and having an allocated person is preferable.

CPR is withheld if the arrest is VT or asystole until shocks have been administered or the external pacing has been commenced, but if this has failed then CPR must be commenced. The person performing CPR will most likely need to be on the opposite side of the table to the cardiologist, and if the table is fairly high they may need a step to stand on. Hands should be linked together and elbow straight and CPR is performed on the lower half of the sternum.

Recommendations	Class	Level
Ventricular fibrillation (VF), pulseless ventricular tachycardia (VT) and asystole may all be diagnosed immediately based on the monitoring in the catheter lab (figure 1). There is no need to routinely look, listen and feel for 10 s.	I	C
Many cases of pulseless electrical activity (PEA) may also be diagnosed by the absence of pulsatile traces but if in doubt then either look, listen and feel or use echocardiography to look for a cardiac output.	IIa	C
If a patient has circulatory collapse with a rate less than 30/min then we define this as extreme bradycardia as this may respond to percussion, external or temporary wire pacing and thus we recommend following the asystole pathway.	I	C
If a patient has an arrhythmia above a rate of 140/min without a discernible cardiac output then we recommend following the pathway for VF/pulseless VT as this may respond to defibrillation.	IIa	C

The general algorithm recommends a depth of 5–6 cm and there are devices available to measure whether you are compressing adequately, but if your patient has an arterial line in place then in fact this can function as a direct measure of the quality of your CPR. In this situation you should compress the chest hard enough that you achieve a systolic pressure of

Dunning J, et al. Heart 2022;0:1–18. doi:10.1136/heartjnl-2021-320588

[6]Anaesthesia and Intensive Care, Southampton University Hospitals NHS Trust, Southampton, UK
[7]Essex Cardiothoracic Centre, Mid and South Essex NHS Trust, Basildon, UK
[8]Medical Technology Research Centre, Anglia Ruskin School of Medicine, Chelmsford, UK
[9]Cardiovascular Care Partnership (UK), British Cardiovascular Society, London, UK
[10]Department of Cardiac Surgery, Royal Sussex County Hospital, Brighton, UK
[11]Department of Cardiothoracic Anaesthesia and Critical Care, Manchester University NHS Foundation Trust, Manchester, UK
[12]Department of Cardiology, Manchester University NHS Foundation Trust, Manchester, UK
[13]School of Healthcare Science, Manchester Metropolitan University, Manchester, UK
[14]Sudden Cardiac Arrest UK, UK

Twitter Nick Curzen @NickCurzen

Acknowledgements The authors thank Dr Piero Farina from the Fondazione Policlinico Universitario 'Agostino Gemelli' IRCCS, in Rome who created the artwork for the Joint societies organisational poster. The authors also thank Sue Hampshire, Director of Clinical Development for the Resuscitation Council UK who guided them through the process of creating this Resuscitation Council approved and NICE accredited guideline.

Contributors All authors contributed to the discussions of the Working Group, the drafting of the document and approved the final version.

Funding The authors have not declared a specific grant for this research from any funding agency in the public, commercial or not-for-profit sectors.

Competing interests JPdB is member of council for the British Heart Rhythm Society, a co-opted member of council for the Resuscitation Council UK, and a practising interventional cardiac electrophysiologist. EG received Abbott Vascular educational funding. SR is a trustee of Heart Valve Voice and Immediate Past President of the British Cardiovascular Society. NO is Immediate Past President for the Association for Cardiothoracic Anaesthesia and Critical Care. CD is on the Executive Committee for the Resuscitation Council UKALS Working Group, ILCOR. JS is lead of a non-profit cardiac catheter laboratory resuscitation educational programme based in Wythenshawe Hospital, Lead Cardiology Clinician, CLEMS course at Wythenshawe Hospital. AA is Vice President for Clinical Standards, British Cardiovascular Society. TK is an advisory board member of the Zoll Medical COOL AMI EU clinical study, received research funds to support cardiac arrest projects from Zoll, and received speaker fees from BD (www.bd.com). JD is co-founder of Cardiac Advanced Resuscitation Education (www.csu-als.org) which is a group that trains clinicians worldwide for emergencies in catheter laboratories, emergencies after cardiac surgery, and thoracic emergency department care. JD is Deputy Editor of www.ctsnet.org, on the SCTS Thoracic Subcommittee, ISMICS Board of Directors 2017, and is STS Workforce Chairman for guideline for resuscitation after cardiac surgery. All other authors declare no competing interests.

Patient and public involvement Patients were involved in the design, conduct, and reporting, with dissemination, and two patients are co-authors of this guideline.

Patient consent for publication Not applicable.

Ethics approval This study does not involve human participants.

Provenance and peer review Commissioned; externally peer reviewed.

ORCID iDs
Joel Dunning http://orcid.org/0000-0001-8792-5089
Andrew Archbold http://orcid.org/0000-0002-9847-070X
Nick Curzen http://orcid.org/0000-0001-9651-7829
Simon Ray http://orcid.org/0000-0001-7775-1900

REFERENCES

1 Webb JG, Solankhi NK, Chugh SK, et al. Incidence, correlates, and outcome of cardiac arrest associated with percutaneous coronary intervention. *Am J Cardiol* 2002;90:1252–4.
2 Mehta RH, Harjai KJ, Grines L, et al. Sustained ventricular tachycardia or fibrillation in the cardiac catheterization laboratory among patients receiving primary percutaneous coronary intervention: incidence, predictors, and outcomes. *J Am Coll Cardiol* 2004;43:1765–72.
3 Sprung J, Ritter MJ, Rihal CS, et al. Outcomes of cardiopulmonary resuscitation and predictors of survival in patients undergoing coronary angiography including percutaneous coronary interventions. *Anesth Analg* 2006;102:217–24.
4 Sinning C, Ahrens I, Cariou A, et al. The cardiac arrest centre for the treatment of sudden cardiac arrest due to presumed cardiac cause: aims, function, and structure: position paper of the ACVC association of the ESC, EAPCI, EHRA, ERC, EUSEM, and ESICM. *Eur Heart J Acute Cardiovasc Care* 2020;34.
5 Soar J, Mitchell S, Gwinnutt C. Resus Council UK. publication: guidelines development process manual. Available: https://www.resus.org.uk/library/publications/publication-guidelines-development-process-manual [Accessed 22 May 2021].
6 European Society of Cardiology. Governing policies and procedures for the writing of ESC clinical practice guidelines, 2017. Available: https://www.escardio.org/static-file/Escardio/Guidelines/About/Recommendations-Guidelines-Production.pdf[Accessed 22 May 2021].
7 Merchant RM, Topjian AA, Panchal AR, et al. Part 1: Executive summary: 2020 American heart association guidelines for cardiopulmonary resuscitation and emergency cardiovascular care. *Circulation* 2020;142:S337–57.
8 Lott C, Truhlář A, Alfonzo A, et al. European resuscitation Council guidelines 2021: cardiac arrest in special circumstances. *Resuscitation* 2021;161:152–219.
9 The Australian and New Zealand Council on Resuscitation. *Resuscitation : A guide for advanced rescuers. Resuscitation in Special Circumstances. Guideline 11*, 2011.
10 Olasveengen TM, Mancini ME, Perkins GD, et al. Adult basic life support: 2020 international consensus on cardiopulmonary resuscitation and emergency cardiovascular care science with treatment recommendations. *Circulation* 2020;142.
11 Gazmuri RJ, Bossaert L, Mosesso V. In adult victims of ventricular fibrillation with long response times, a period of CPR before attempting defibrillation may improve ROSC and survival to hospital discharge. W68 and W177: appendix. *Circulation* 2005.
12 Wik L, Hansen TB, Fylling F, et al. Delaying defibrillation to give basic cardiopulmonary resuscitation to patients with out-of-hospital ventricular fibrillation: a randomized trial. *JAMA* 2003;289:1389–95.
13 Jacobs IG, Finn JC, Oxer HF, et al. Cpr before defibrillation in out-of-hospital cardiac arrest: a randomized trial. *Emerg Med Australas* 2005;17:39–45.
14 Cobb LA, Fahrenbruch CE, Walsh TR, et al. Influence of cardiopulmonary resuscitation prior to defibrillation in patients with out-of-hospital ventricular fibrillation. *JAMA* 1999;281:1182–8.
15 Stotz M, Albrecht R, Zwicker G, et al. Ems defibrillation-first policy may not improve outcome in out-of-hospital cardiac arrest. *Resuscitation* 2003;58:277–82.
16 Chan PS, Krumholz HM, Nichol G, et al. Delayed time to defibrillation after in-hospital cardiac arrest. *N Engl J Med* 2008;358:9–17.
17 Spearpoint KG, McLean CP, Zideman DA. Early defibrillation and the chain of survival in 'in-hospital' adult cardiac arrest; minutes count. *Resuscitation* 2000;44:165–9.
18 Richardson L, Dissanayake A, Dunning J. What cardioversion protocol for ventricular fibrillation should be followed for patients who arrest shortly post-cardiac surgery? *Interact Cardiovasc Thorac Surg* 2007;6:799–805.
19 Lockowandt U, Levine A, Strang T, et al. If a patient arrests after cardiac surgery is it acceptable to delay cardiopulmonary resuscitation until you have attempted either defibrillation or pacing? *Interact Cardiovasc Thorac Surg* 2008;7:878–85.
20 Link MS, Berkow LC, Kudenchuk PJ, et al. Part 7: adult advanced cardiovascular life support: 2015 American heart association guidelines update for cardiopulmonary resuscitation and emergency cardiovascular care. *Circulation* 2015;132:S444–64.
21 Dee R, Smith M, Rajendran K, et al. The effect of alternative methods of cardiopulmonary resuscitation - Cough CPR, percussion pacing or precordial thump - on outcomes following cardiac arrest. A systematic review. *Resuscitation* 2021;162:73–81.
22 Niemann JT, Rosborough J, Hausknecht M, et al. Cough-CPR: documentation of systemic perfusion in man and in an experimental model: a "window" to the mechanism of blood flow in external CPR. *Crit Care Med* 1980;8:141–6.
23 Saba SE, David SW. Sustained consciousness during ventricular fibrillation: case report of cough cardiopulmonary resuscitation. *Cathet Cardiovasc Diagn* 1996;37:47–8.
24 Miller B, Cohen A, Serio A, et al. Hemodynamics of cough cardiopulmonary resuscitation in a patient with sustained torsades de pointes/ventricular flutter. *J Emerg Med* 1994;12:627–32.
25 Criley JM, Blaufuss AH, Kissel GL. Cough-Induced cardiac compression. self-administered from of cardiopulmonary resuscitation. *JAMA* 1976;236:1246–50.
26 Klumbies A, Paliege R, Volkmann H. Mechanische Notfallstimulation bei Asystolie und extremer Bradykardie [Mechanical emergency stimulation in asystole and extreme bradycardia]. *Z Gesamte Inn Med* 1988;43:348–52.
27 Zeh E, Rahner E. Die manuelle extrathorakale Stimulation des Herzens. Zur Technik und Wirkung des "Präkordialschlages" [The manual extrathoracal stimulation of the heart. Technique and effect of the precordial thump (author's transl)]. *Z Kardiol* 1978;67:299–304.
28 Ramirez FD, Sadek MM, Boileau I, et al. Evaluation of a novel cardioversion intervention for atrial fibrillation: the Ottawa AF cardioversion protocol. *Europace* 2019;21:708–15.
29 January CT, Wann LS, et al. 2014 AHA/ACC/HRS guideline for the management of patients with atrial fibrillation: a report of the American College of Cardiology/American heart association Task force on practice guidelines and the heart rhythm Society. *Circulation* 2014;130.
30 Kerber RE, Grayzel J, Hoyt R, et al. Transthoracic resistance in human defibrillation. Influence of body weight, chest size, serial shocks, paddle size and paddle contact pressure. *Circulation* 1981;63:676–82.
31 Sima SJ, Ferguson DW, Charbonnier F, et al. Factors affecting transthoracic impedance during electrical cardioversion. *Am J Cardiol* 1988;62:1048–52.

32 Ramirez FD, Fiset SL, Cleland MJ, et al. Effect of applying force to Self-Adhesive electrodes on transthoracic impedance: implications for electrical cardioversion. Pacing Clin Electrophysiol 2016;39:1141–7.

33 Olasveengen TM, Wik L, Sunde K, et al. Outcome when adrenaline (epinephrine) was actually given vs. not given - post hoc analysis of a randomized clinical trial. Resuscitation 2012;83:327–32.

34 Lin S, Callaway CW, Shah PS, et al. Adrenaline for out-of-hospital cardiac arrest resuscitation: a systematic review and meta-analysis of randomized controlled trials. Resuscitation 2014;85:732–40.

35 Perkins GD, Ji C, Deakin CD, et al. A randomized trial of epinephrine in out-of-hospital cardiac arrest. N Engl J Med 2018;379:711–21.

36 Addala S, Kahn JK, Moccia TF, et al. Outcome of ventricular fibrillation developing during percutaneous coronary interventions in 19,497 patients without cardiogenic shock. Am J Cardiol 2005;96:764–5.

37 Tavakol M, Ashraf S, Brener SJ. Risks and complications of coronary angiography: a comprehensive review. Glob J Health Sci 2012;4:65–93.

38 Al-Hijji MA, Lennon RJ, Gulati R, et al. Safety and risk of major complications with diagnostic cardiac catheterization. Circ Cardiovasc Interv 2019;12:e007791.

39 Wagner H, Rundgren M, Hardig BM. A structured approach for treatment of prolonged cardiac arrest cases in the coronary catheterization laboratory using mechanical chest compressions. Int J Cardiovasc Res 2018;2:4.

40 Sutton RM, French B, Meaney PA, et al. Physiologic monitoring of CPR quality during adult cardiac arrest: a propensity-matched cohort study. Resuscitation 2016;106:76–82.

41 Kinnaird T, Kwok CS, Davies R. British cardiovascular intervention Society and the National Institute for cardiovascular outcomes research. coronary perforation complicating percutaneous coronary intervention in patients presenting with an acute coronary syndrome: an analysis of 1013 perforation cases from the British cardiovascular intervention Society database. Int J Cardiol 2020;299:37–4235.

42 Chalkias A, Arnaoutoglou E, Xanthos T. Personalized physiology-guided resuscitation in highly monitored patients with cardiac arrest-the PERSEUS resuscitation protocol. Heart Fail Rev 2019;24:473–80.

43 Corral Torres E, Hernández-Tejedor A, Suárez Bustamante R, et al. Prognostic value of venous blood analysis at the start of CPR in non-traumatic out-of-hospital cardiac arrest: association with ROSC and the neurological outcome. Crit Care 2020;24:60.

44 Chopra AS, Wong N, Ziegler CP, et al. Systematic review and meta-analysis of hemodynamic-directed feedback during cardiopulmonary resuscitation in cardiac arrest. Resuscitation 2016;101:102–7.

45 Kudenchuk PJ, Cobb LA, Copass MK, et al. Amiodarone for resuscitation after out-of-hospital cardiac arrest due to ventricular fibrillation. N Engl J Med 1999;341:871–8.

46 Dorian P, Cass D, Schwartz B, et al. Amiodarone as compared with lidocaine for shock-resistant ventricular fibrillation. N Engl J Med 2002;346:884–90.

47 Kudenchuk PJ, Brown SP, Daya M, et al. Resuscitation outcomes Consortium-Amiodarone, lidocaine or placebo study (ROC-ALPS): rationale and methodology behind an out-of-hospital cardiac arrest antiarrhythmic drug trial. Am Heart J 2014;167:653-9.e4.

48 Kudenchuk PJ, Brown SP, Daya M, et al. Amiodarone, lidocaine, or placebo in out-of-hospital cardiac arrest. N Engl J Med 2016;374:1711–22.

49 Cave DM, Gazmuri RJ, Otto CW, et al. Part 7: CPR techniques and devices: 2010 American heart association guidelines for cardiopulmonary resuscitation and emergency cardiovascular care. Circulation 2010;122:S720–8.

50 Clattenburg EJ, Wroe PC, Gardner K, et al. Implementation of the cardiac arrest sonographic assessment (CASA) protocol for patients with cardiac arrest is associated with shorter CPR pulse checks. Resuscitation 2018;131:69–73.

51 Parker BK, Salerno A, Euerle BD. The use of transesophageal echocardiography during cardiac arrest resuscitation: a literature review. J Ultrasound Med 2019;38:1141–51.

52 Andros G, Harris RW, Dulawa LB, et al. Subclavian artery catheterization: a new approach for endovascular procedures. J Vasc Surg 1994;20:566–76.

53 Park GY, JH O, Yoon Y. J Korean fluoroscopy guided percutaneous catheter drainage of pneumothorax in patients with failed chest tube drainage. Radiol Soc 1995;33:889–92.

54 Hallstrom A, Rea TD, Sayre MR, et al. Manual chest compression vs use of an automated chest compression device during resuscitation following out-of-hospital cardiac arrest: a randomized trial. JAMA 2006;295:2620–8.

55 Wik L, Olsen J-A, Persse D, et al. Manual vs. integrated automatic load-distributing band CPR with equal survival after out of hospital cardiac arrest. The randomized CIRC trial. Resuscitation 2014;85:741–8.

56 Brooks SC, Hassan N, Bigham BL, et al. Mechanical versus manual chest compressions for cardiac arrest. Cochrane Database Syst Rev 2014:CD007260.

57 The AutoPulse non-invasive cardiac support pump for cardiopulmonary resuscitation Medtech innovation briefing published: 12 February 2015 by the National Institute for health and care excellence. Available: nice.org.uk/guidance/mib18

58 Wang PL, Brooks SC, Cochrane Heart Group. Mechanical versus manual chest compressions for cardiac arrest. Cochrane Database Syst Rev 2018;16:CD007260.

59 Couper K, Yeung J, Nicholson T, et al. Mechanical chest compression devices at in-hospital cardiac arrest: a systematic review and meta-analysis. Resuscitation 2016;103:24–31.

60 Gates S, Quinn T, Deakin CD, et al. Mechanical chest compression for out of hospital cardiac arrest: systematic review and meta-analysis. Resuscitation 2015;94:91–7.

61 Esibov A, Banville I, Chapman FW, et al. Mechanical chest compressions improved aspects of CPR in the LINc trial. Resuscitation 2015;91:116–21.

62 Grogaard HK, Wik L, Eriksen M, et al. Continuous mechanical chest compressions during cardiac arrest to facilitate restoration of coronary circulation with percutaneous coronary intervention. J Am Coll Cardiol 2007;50:1093–4.

63 Agostoni P, Cornelis K, Vermeersch P. Successful percutaneous treatment of an intraprocedural left main stent thrombosis with the support of an automatic mechanical chest compression device. Int J Cardiol 2008;124:e19–21.

64 Steen S, Sjöberg T, Olsson P, et al. Treatment of out-of-hospital cardiac arrest with LUCAS, a new device for automatic mechanical compression and active decompression resuscitation. Resuscitation 2005;67:25–30.

65 Larsen AI, Hjørnevik AS, Ellingsen CL, et al. Cardiac arrest with continuous mechanical chest compression during percutaneous coronary intervention. A report on the use of the LUCAS device. Resuscitation 2007;75:454–9.

66 Wagner H, Terkelsen CJ, Friberg H, et al. Cardiac arrest in the catheterisation laboratory: a 5-year experience of using mechanical chest compressions to facilitate PCI during prolonged resuscitation efforts. Resuscitation 2010;81:383–7.

67 Libungan B, Dworeck C, Omerovic E. Successful percutaneous coronary intervention during cardiac arrest with use of an automated chest compression device: a case report. Ther Clin Risk Manag 2014;10:255–7.

68 Stub D, Bernard S, Pellegrino V, et al. Refractory cardiac arrest treated with mechanical CPR, hypothermia, ECMO and early reperfusion (the CHEER trial). Resuscitation 2015;86:88–94.

69 Levy M, Yost D, Walker RG, et al. A quality improvement initiative to optimize use of a mechanical chest compression device within a high-performance CPR approach to out-of-hospital cardiac arrest resuscitation. Resuscitation 2015;92:32-7.

70 Couper K, Velho RM, Quinn T, et al. Training approaches for the deployment of a mechanical chest compression device: a randomised controlled manikin study. BMJ Open 2018;8:e019009.

71 Yannopoulos D, Bartos J, Raveendran G, et al. Advanced reperfusion strategies for patients with out-of-hospital cardiac arrest and refractory ventricular fibrillation (arrest): a phase 2, single centre, open-label, randomised controlled trial. Lancet 2020;396:1807–16.

72 Ladowski JS, Dillon TA, Deschner WP, et al. Durability of emergency coronary artery bypass for complications of failed angioplasty. Cardiovasc Surg 1996;4:23–7.

73 Redle J, King B, Lemole G, et al. Utility of rapid percutaneous cardiopulmonary bypass for refractory hemodynamic collapse in the cardiac catheterization laboratory. Am J Cardiol 1994;73:899–900.

74 Overlie PA. Emergency use of portable cardiopulmonary bypass. Cathet Cardiovasc Diagn 1990;20:27–31.

75 Shawl FA, Domanski MJ, Wish MH, et al. Emergency cardiopulmonary bypass support in patients with cardiac arrest in the catheterization laboratory. Cathet Cardiovasc Diagn 1990;19:8–12.

76 Bagai J, Webb D, Kasasbeh E, et al. Efficacy and safety of percutaneous life support during high-risk percutaneous coronary intervention, refractory cardiogenic shock and in-laboratory cardiopulmonary arrest. J Invasive Cardiol 2011;23:141–7.

77 Sheu J-J, Tsai T-H, Lee F-Y, et al. Early extracorporeal membrane oxygenator-assisted primary percutaneous coronary intervention improved 30-day clinical outcomes in patients with ST-segment elevation myocardial infarction complicated with profound cardiogenic shock. Crit Care Med 2010;38:1810–7.

78 Arlt M, Philipp A, Voelkel S, et al. Early experiences with miniaturized extracorporeal life-support in the catheterization laboratory. Eur J Cardiothorac Surg 2012;42:858–63.

79 Huang C-C, Hsu J-C, Wu Y-W, et al. Implementation of extracorporeal membrane oxygenation before primary percutaneous coronary intervention may improve the survival of patients with ST-segment elevation myocardial infarction and refractory cardiogenic shock. Int J Cardiol 2018;269:45–50.

80 van den Brink FS, Magan AD, Noordzij PG, et al. Veno-Arterial extracorporeal membrane oxygenation in addition to primary PCI in patients presenting with ST-elevation myocardial infarction. Neth Heart J 2018;26:76–84.

81 Abrams D, Garan AR, Abdelbary A, et al. Position paper for the organization of ECMO programs for cardiac failure in adults. Intensive Care Med 2018;44:717–29.

82 Thiele H, Zeymer U, Neumann F-J, et al. Intra-Aortic balloon counterpulsation in acute myocardial infarction complicated by cardiogenic shock (IABP-SHOCK II): final 12 month results of a randomised, open-label trial. Lancet 2013;382:1638–45.

83 Ohman EM, George BS, White CJ, et al. Use of aortic counterpulsation to improve sustained coronary artery patency during acute myocardial infarction. Results of a randomized trial. The randomized IABP Study Group. Circulation 1994;90:792–9.

84 Kaul U, Sahay S, Bahl VK, et al. Coronary angioplasty in high risk patients: comparison of elective intraaortic balloon pump and percutaneous cardiopulmonary bypass support--a randomized study. J Interv Cardiol 1995;8:199–205.

85 Stone GW, Marsalese D, Brodie BR, et al. A prospective, randomized evaluation of prophylactic intraaortic balloon counterpulsation in high risk patients with acute myocardial infarction treated with primary angioplasty. second primary angioplasty in myocardial infarction (PAMI-II) trial Investigators. J Am Coll Cardiol 1997;29:1459–67.

Guideline or consensus statement

86 Ohman EM, Nanas J, Stomel RJ, et al. Thrombolysis and counterpulsation to improve survival in myocardial infarction complicated by hypotension and suspected cardiogenic shock or heart failure: results of the tactics trial. J Thromb Thrombolysis 2005;19:33–9.

87 Prondzinsky R, Lemm H, Swyter M, et al. Intra-Aortic balloon counterpulsation in patients with acute myocardial infarction complicated by cardiogenic shock: the prospective, randomized IABP shock trial for attenuation of multiorgan dysfunction syndrome. Crit Care Med 2010;38:152–60.

88 Unverzagt S, Buerke M, de Waha A, et al. Intra-Aortic balloon pump counterpulsation (IABP) for myocardial infarction complicated by cardiogenic shock. Cochrane Database Syst Rev 2015:CD007398.

89 Sjauw KD, Engström AE, Vis MM, et al. A systematic review and meta-analysis of intra-aortic balloon pump therapy in ST-elevation myocardial infarction: should we change the guidelines? Eur Heart J 2009;30:459-68.

90 Lee JM, Park J, Kang J, et al. The efficacy and safety of mechanical hemodynamic support in patients undergoing high-risk percutaneous coronary intervention with or without cardiogenic shock: Bayesian approach network meta-analysis of 13 randomized controlled trials. Int J Cardiol 2015;184:36–46.

91 Firdaus I, Yuniadi Y, Andriantoro H, et al. Early insertion of intra-aortic balloon pump after cardiac arrest on acute coronary syndrome patients: a randomized clinical trial. Cardiol Cardiovasc Med 2019;03:193–203.

92 Iqbal MB, Al-Hussaini A, Rosser G, et al. Intra-Aortic balloon pump counterpulsation in the post-resuscitation period is associated with improved functional outcomes in patients surviving an out-of-hospital cardiac arrest: insights from a dedicated heart attack centre. Heart Lung Circ 2016;25:1210–7.

93 Emerman CL, Pinchak AC, Hagen JF, et al. Hemodynamic effects of the intra-aortic balloon pump during experimental cardiac arrest. Am J Emerg Med 1989;7:378–83.

94 Vase H, Christensen S, Christiansen A, et al. The Impella CP device for acute mechanical circulatory support in refractory cardiac arrest. Resuscitation 2017;112:70–4.

95 Kamran H, Batra S, Venesy DM, et al. Outcomes of Impella CP insertion during cardiac arrest: a single center experience. Resuscitation 2020;147:53–6.

96 Panagides V, Vase H, Shah SP, et al. Impella CP implantation during cardiopulmonary resuscitation for cardiac arrest: a multicenter experience. J Clin Med 2021;10:339.

97 Dimas VV, Morray BH, Kim DW, et al. A multicenter study of the impella device for mechanical support of the systemic circulation in pediatric and adolescent patients. Catheter Cardiovasc Interv 2017;90:124–9.

98 Henriques JP, Remmelink M, JJr B. Safety and feasibility of elective high-risk percutaneous coronary intervention procedures with left ventricular support of the Impella recover Lp 2.5. Am J Cardiol 2006.

99 Sjauw KD, Konorza T, Erbel R, et al. Supported high-risk percutaneous coronary intervention with the Impella 2.5 device the Europella registry. J Am Coll Cardiol 2009;54:2430–4.

100 Vecchio S, Chechi T, Giuliani G, et al. Use of Impella recover 2.5 left ventricular assist device in patients with cardiogenic shock or undergoing high-risk percutaneous coronary intervention procedures: experience of a high-volume center. Minerva Cardioangiol 2008;56:391–9.

101 Udesen NJ, Møller JE, Lindholm MG, et al. Rationale and design of danger shock: Danish-German cardiogenic shock trial. Am Heart J 2019;214:60–8.

102 Sethi A, Singbal Y, Kodumuri V, et al. Inpatient mortality and its predictors after pericardiocentesis: an analysis from the nationwide inpatient sample 2009-2013. J Interv Cardiol 2018;31:815–25.

103 Tsang TSM, Enriquez-Sarano M, Freeman WK, et al. Consecutive 1127 therapeutic echocardiographically guided pericardiocenteses: clinical profile, practice patterns, and outcomes spanning 21 years. Mayo Clin Proc 2002;77:429–36.

104 Cho BC, Kang SM, Kim DH, et al. Clinical and echocardiographic characteristics of pericardial effusion in patients who underwent echocardiographically guided pericardiocentesis: Yonsei cardiovascular center experience, 1993-2003. Yonsei Med J 2004;45:462–8.

105 Ristić AD, Imazio M, Adler Y, et al. Triage strategy for urgent management of cardiac tamponade: a position statement of the European Society of cardiology Working group on myocardial and pericardial diseases. Eur Heart J 2014;35:2279-84.

106 Kinnaird T, Kwok CS, Kontopantelis E. An analysis of 527 121 cases from the British cardiovascular intervention Society database. Circ Cardiovasc Interv 2016;9:e003449.

107 Ellis SG, Ajluni S, Arnold AZ, et al. Increased coronary perforation in the new device era. incidence, classification, management, and outcome. Circulation 1994;90:2725–30.

108 Hsu JC, Varosy PD, Bao H, et al. Cardiac perforation from implantable cardioverter-defibrillator lead placement: insights from the National cardiovascular data registry. Circ Cardiovasc Qual Outcomes 2013;6:582–90.

109 Joseph De Bono on Behlaf of the British Heart Rhythm Society Council April. Standards for interventional electrophysiology study and catheter ablation in adults, 2020. Available: https://bhrs.com/wp-content/uploads/2020/04/British-Heart-Rhythm-Society-Standards-Ablation-2020-1.pdf

110 Konstantinides SV, Torbicki A, Agnelli G. 2014 ESC guidelines on the diagnosis and management of acute pulmonary embolism. Eur Heart J 2014;35.

111 Bergum D, Nordseth T, Mjølstad OC, et al. Causes of in-hospital cardiac arrest - incidences and rate of recognition. Resuscitation 2015;87:63–8.

112 Kürkciyan I, Meron G, Sterz F, et al. Pulmonary embolism as a cause of cardiac arrest: presentation and outcome. Arch Intern Med 2000;160:1529–35.

113 MacCarthy P, Worrall A, McCarthy G, et al. The use of transthoracic echocardiography to guide thrombolytic therapy during cardiac arrest due to massive pulmonary embolism. Emerg Med J 2002;19:178–9.

114 Aagaard R, Caap P, Hansson NC, et al. Detection of pulmonary embolism during cardiac Arrest-Ultrasonographic findings should be interpreted with caution. Crit Care Med 2017;45:e695–702.

115 Li X, Fu Q-ling, Jing X-li, et al. A meta-analysis of cardiopulmonary resuscitation with and without the administration of thrombolytic agents. Resuscitation 2006;70:31–6.

116 Böttiger BW, Arntz H-R, Chamberlain DA, et al. Thrombolysis during resuscitation for out-of-hospital cardiac arrest. N Engl J Med 2008;359:2651–62.

117 Javaudin F, Lascarrou J-B, Le Bastard Q, et al. Thrombolysis During Resuscitation for Out-of-Hospital Cardiac Arrest Caused by Pulmonary Embolism Increases 30-Day Survival: Findings From the French National Cardiac Arrest Registry. Chest 2019;156:1167–75.

118 Javaudin F, Lascarrou J-B, Esquina H, et al. Improving identification of pulmonary embolism-related out-of-hospital cardiac arrest to optimize thrombolytic therapy during resuscitation. Crit Care 2019;23:409.

119 Konstantinides SV, Meyer G. The 2019 ESC guidelines on the diagnosis and management of acute pulmonary embolism. Eur Heart J 2019;40:3453–5.

120 Alqahtani F, Munir MB, Aljohani S, et al. Surgical thrombectomy for pulmonary embolism: updated performance rates and outcomes. Tex Heart Inst J 2019;46:172–4.

121 Rousseau H, Del Giudice C, Sanchez O, et al. Endovascular therapies for pulmonary embolism. Heliyon 2021;7:e06574.

122 O'Malley TJ, Choi JH, Maynes EJ, et al. Outcomes of extracorporeal life support for the treatment of acute massive pulmonary embolism: a systematic review. Resuscitation 2020;146:132–7.

123 Fava M, Loyola S, Bertoni H, et al. Massive pulmonary embolism: percutaneous mechanical thrombectomy during cardiopulmonary resuscitation. J Vasc Interv Radiol 2005;16:119–23.

124 Dankiewicz J, Cronberg T, Lilja G, et al. Hypothermia versus normothermia after out-of-hospital cardiac arrest. N Engl J Med 2021;384:2283–94.

125 Nolan JP, Sandroni C, Böttiger BW, et al. European resuscitation Council and European Society of intensive care medicine guidelines 2021: post-resuscitation care. Intensive Care Med 2021;47:369–421.

126 Greif R, Bhanji F, Bigham BL, et al. Education, implementation, and teams: 2020 international consensus on cardiopulmonary resuscitation and emergency cardiovascular care science with treatment recommendations. Resuscitation 2020;156:A188–239.

Notes

1.   Lin S, Callaway CW, Shah PS, et al. Adrenaline for out-of-hospital cardiac arrest resuscitation: a systematic review and meta-analysis of randomized controlled trials. Resuscitation 2014; 85: 732-40.

2.   G.D. Perkins, C. Ji, C.D. Deakin, T. Quinn, J.P. Nolan, C. Scomparin, S. Regan, J. Long, A. Slowther, H. Pocock, J.J.M. Black, F. Moore, R.T. Fothergill, N. Rees, L. O'Shea, M. Docherty, I. Gunson, K. Han, K. Charlton, J. Finn, S. Petrou,N. Stallard, S. Gates, and R. Lall, for the PARAMEDIC2 Collaborators*. A Randomized Trial of Epinephrine in Out-of-Hospital Cardiac Arrest, The New England Journal of Medicine, July 22, 2018 , DOI: 10.1056/NEJMoa1806842

3.   Webb JG, Solankhi NK, Chugh SK, Amin H, Buller CE, Ricci DR, Humphries K, Penn IM, Carere R. Incidence, correlates, and outcome of cardiac arrest associated with percutaneous coronary intervention. Am J Cardiol. 2002;90:1252–1254.

4.   Mehta RH, Harjai KJ, Grines L, Stone GW, Boura J, Cox D, O'Neill W, Grines CL; Primary Angioplasty in Myocardial Infarction (PAMI) Investigators. Sustained ventricular tachycardia or fibrillation in the cardiac catheterization laboratory among patients receiving primary percutaneous coronary intervention: incidence, predictors, and outcomes. J Am Coll Cardiol. 2004;43:1765–1772. doi:10.1016/j.jacc.2003.09.072.

5.   Martin-Yuste V, Alvarez-Contreras L, Brugaletta S, Ferreira-Gonzalez I, Cola C, Garcia-Picart J, Martí V, Sabate M. Emergent versus elective percutaneous stent implantation in the unprotected left main: long-term outcomes from a single-center registry. J Invasive Cardiol. 2011;23:392–397.

6.   Sprung J, Ritter MJ, Rihal CS, Warner ME, Wilson GA, Williams BA, Stevens SR, Schroeder DR, Bourke DL, Warner DO. Outcomes of cardiopulmonary resuscitation and predictors of survival in patients undergoing coronary angiography including percutaneous coronary interventions. Anesth Analg. 2006;102:217–224. doi: 10.1213/01.ane.0000189082.54614.26.

7.   Addala S, Kahn JK, Moccia TF, Harjai K, Pellizon G, Ochoa A, O'Neill WW. Outcome of ventricular fibrillation developing during percutaneous coronary interventions in 19,497 patients without
        cardiogenic shock. Am Cardiol. 2005;96:764–765. doi: 10.1016/j.amjcard.2005.04.057.

8.   O'Gara PT, Kushner FG, Ascheim DD, Casey DE Jr, Chung MK, de Lemos JA, Ettinger SM, Fang JC, Fesmire FM, Franklin BA, Granger CB, Krumholz HM, Linderbaum JA, Morrow DA, Newby LK, Ornato JP, Ou N, Radford MJ, Tamis-Holland JE, Tommaso CL, Tracy CM, Woo YJ, Zhao DX. 2013 ACCF/AHA guideline for the management of ST-elevation myocardial infarction: a report of the
        American College of Cardiology Foundation/American Heart Association Task Force on Practice Guidelines. Circulation. 2013;127:e362–e425. doi: 10.1161/CIR.0b013e3182742cf6.

9.   Grogaard HK, Wik L, Eriksen M, Brekke M, Sunde K. Continuous mechanical chest compressions during cardiac arrest to facilitate restoration of coronary circulation with percutaneous coronary intervention. J Am Coll Cardiol. 2007;50:1093–1094. doi: 10.1016/j.

jacc.2007.05.028.

10.   Agostoni P, Cornelis K, Vermeersch P. Successful percutaneous treatment of an intraprocedural left main stent thrombosis with the support of an automatic mechanical chest compression device. Int J Cardiol. 2008;124:e19–e21. doi: 10.1016/j.ijcard.2006.11.175.

11.   Steen S, Sjöberg T, Olsson P, Young M. Treatment of out-of-hospital cardiac arrest with LUCAS, a new device for automatic mechanical compression and active decompression resuscitation. Resuscitation. 2005;67:25–30. doi: 10.1016/j.resuscitation.2005.05.013.

12.   Larsen AI, Hjørnevik AS, Ellingsen CL, Nilsen DW. Cardiac arrest with continuous mechanical chest compression during percutaneous coronary intervention. A report on the use of the LUCAS device. Resuscitation. 2007;75:454–459. doi: 10.1016/j.resuscitation.2007.05.007.

13.   Wagner H, Terkelsen CJ, Friberg H, Harnek J, Kern K, Lassen JF, Olivecrona GK. Cardiac arrest in the catheterisation laboratory: a 5-year experience of using mechanical chest compressions to facilitate PCI during prolonged resuscitation efforts. Resuscitation. 2010;81:383–387. doi: 10.1016/j.resuscitation.2009.11.006.

14.   Linder R, Abdollahi P, Wennersten G. [Life-saving mechanical compression during percutaneous coronary intervention]. Lakartidningen. 2006;103:2390–2392.

15.   Ladowski JS, Dillon TA, Deschner WP, DeRiso AJ 2nd, Peterson AC, Schatzlein MH. Durability of emergency coronary artery bypass for complications of failed angioplasty. Cardiovasc Surg. 1996;4:23–27.

16.   Redle J, King B, Lemole G, Doorey AJ. Utility of rapid percutaneous cardiopulmonary bypass for refractory hemodynamic collapse in the cardiac catheterization laboratory. Am J Cardiol. 1994;73:899–900.

17.   Overlie PA. Emergency use of portable cardiopulmonary bypass. Cathet Cardiovasc Diagn. 1990;20:27–31.

18.   Shawl FA, Domanski MJ, Wish MH, Davis M, Punja S, Hernandez TJ. Emergency cardiopulmonary bypass support in patients with cardiac arrest in the catheterization laboratory. Cathet Cardiovasc Diagn. 1990;19:8–12.

19.   Bagai J, Webb D, Kasasbeh E, Crenshaw M, Salloum J, Chen J, Zhao D. Efficacy and safety of percutaneous life support during high-risk percutaneous coronary intervention, refractory cardiogenic shock and in-laboratory cardiopulmonary arrest. J Invasive Cardiol. 2011;23:141–147.

20.   Sheu JJ, Tsai TH, Lee FY, Fang HY, Sun CK, Leu S, Yang CH, Chen SM, Hang CL, Hsieh YK, Chen CJ, Wu CJ, Yip HK. Early extracorporeal membrane oxygenator-assisted primary percutaneous coronary intervention improved 30-day clinical outcomes in patients with ST-segment elevation myocardial infarction complicated with profound cardiogenic shock. Crit Care Med. 2010;38:1810–1817. doi: 10.1097/CCM.0b013e3181e8acf7.

21.   Arlt M, Philipp A, Voelkel S, Schopka S, Husser O, Hengstenberg C, Schmid C, Hilker M. Early experiences with miniaturized extracorporeal life-support in the catheterization laboratory. Eur J Cardiothorac Surg. 2012;42:858–863. doi: 10.1093/ejcts/ezs176.

22.   Grambow DW, Deeb GM, Pavlides GS, Margulis A, O'Neill WW, Bates ER. Emergent percutaneous cardiopulmonary bypass in patients having cardiovascular collapse in the cardiac catheterization laboratory. Am J Cardiol. 1994;73:872–875.

23.   Mooney MR, Arom KV, Joyce LD, Mooney JF, Goldenberg IF, Von Rueden TJ, Emery RW. Emergency cardiopulmonary bypass support in patients with cardiac arrest. J Thorac Cardiovasc Surg.1991;101:450–454.

24.   Tsao NW, Shih CM, Yeh JS, Kao YT, Hsieh MH, Ou KL, Chen JW, Shyu KG, Weng ZC, Chang NC, Lin FY, Huang CY.Extracorporeal membrane oxygenation-assisted primary percutaneous coronary intervention may improve survival of patients with acute myocardial infarction complicated by profound cardiogenic shock.J Crit Care. 2012; 27:530.e1–530.11. doi: 10.1016/j.jcrc.2012.02.012.CrossrefGoogle Scholar

25.   Thiele H, Zeymer U, Neumann FJ, Ferenc M, Olbrich HG, Hausleiter J, de Waha A, Richardt G, Hennersdorf M, Empen K, Fuernau G, Desch S, Eitel I, Hambrecht R, Lauer B, Böhm M, Ebelt H, Schneider S, Werdan K, Schuler G; Intraaortic Balloon Pump in cardiogenic shock II (IABP-SHOCK II) trial investigators. Intra-aortic balloon counterpulsation in acute myocardial infarction complicated by cardiogenic shock (IABP-SHOCK II): final 12 month results of a randomised, open-label trial.Lancet. 2013; 382:1638–1645. doi: 10.1016/S0140-6736(13)61783-3. CrossrefMedlineGoogle Scholar

26.   Ohman EM, George BS, White CJ, Kern MJ, Gurbel PA, Freedman RJ, Lundergan C, Hartmann JR, Talley JD, Frey MJ.Use of aortic counterpulsation to improve sustained coronary artery patency during acute myocardial infarction. Results of a randomized trial. The Randomized IABP Study Group.Circulation. 1994; 90:792–799.LinkGoogle Scholar

27.   Kaul U, Sahay S, Bahl VK, Sharma S, Wasir HS, Venugopal P.Coronary angioplasty in high risk patients: comparison of elective intraaortic balloon pump and percutaneous cardiopulmonary bypass support–a randomized study.J Interv Cardiol. 1995; 8:199–205.CrossrefMedlineGoogle Scholar

180.   Stone GW, Marsalese D, Brodie BR, Griffin JJ, Donohue B, Costantini C, Balestrini C, Wharton T, Esente P, Spain M, Moses J, Nobuyoshi M, Ayres M, Jones D, Mason D, Grines L, O'Neill WW, Grines CL.A prospective, randomized evaluation of prophylactic intraaortic balloon counterpulsation in high risk patients with acute myocardial infarction treated with primary angioplasty. Second Primary Angioplasty in Myocardial Infarction (PAMI-II) Trial Investigators.J Am Coll Cardiol. 1997; 29:1459–1467.MedlineGoogle Scholar

28.   Ohman EM, Nanas J, Stomel RJ, Leesar MA, Nielsen DW, O'Dea D, Rogers FJ, Harber D, Hudson MP, Fraulo E, Shaw LK, Lee KL; TACTICS Trial. Thrombolysis and counterpulsation to improve survival in myocardial infarction complicated by hypotension and suspected cardiogenic shock or heart failure: results of the TACTICS Trial.J Thromb Thrombolysis. 2005; 19:33–39. doi: 10.1007/s11239-005-0938-0.CrossrefMedlineGoogle Scholar

29.   Prondzinsky R, Lemm H, Swyter M, Wegener N, Unverzagt S, Carter JM, Russ M, Schlitt A, Buerke U, Christoph A, Schmidt H, Winkler M, Thiery J, Werdan K, Buerke M.Intra-aortic balloon counterpulsation in patients with acute myocardial infarction complicated by cardiogenic shock: the prospective, randomized IABP SHOCK Trial for attenuation of multiorgan dysfunction syndrome.Crit Care Med. 2010; 38:152–160. doi: 10.1097/CCM.0b013e3181b78671. CrossrefMedlineGoogle Scholar

30.   Unverzagt S, Buerke M, de Waha A, Haerting J, Pietzner D, Seyfarth M, Thiele H, Werdan K, Zeymer U, Prondzinsky R.Intra-aortic balloon pump counterpulsation (IABP) for myocardi-

al infarction complicated by cardiogenic shock.Cochrane Database Syst Rev. 2015; 3:CD007398. doi: 10.1002/14651858.CD007398.pub3.Google Scholar

31.   Sjauw KD, Engström AE, Vis MM, van der Schaaf RJ, Baan J, Koch KT, de Winter RJ, Piek JJ, Tijssen JG, Henriques JP.A systematic review and meta-analysis of intra-aortic balloon pump therapy in ST-elevation myocardial infarction: should we change the guidelines?Eur Heart J. 2009; 30:459–468. doi: 10.1093/eurheartj/ehn602.CrossrefMedlineGoogle Scholar

32.   Lee JM, Park J, Kang J, Jeon KH, Jung JH, Lee SE, Han JK, Kim HL, Yang HM, Park KW, Kang HJ, Koo BK, Kim SH, Kim HS.The efficacy and safety of mechanical hemodynamic support in patients undergoing high-risk percutaneous coronary intervention with or without cardiogenic shock: Bayesian approach network meta-analysis of 13 randomized controlled trials.Int J Cardiol. 2015; 184:36–46. doi: 10.1016/j.ijcard.2015.01.081.CrossrefMedlineGoogle Scholar

33.   Reul GJ, Cooley DA, Hallman GL, Duncan JM, Livesay JJ, Frazier OH, Ott DA, Angelini P, Massumi A, Mathur VS.Coronary artery bypass for unsuccessful percutaneous transluminal coronary angioplasty.J Thorac Cardiovasc Surg. 1984; 88(5 Pt 1):685–694.CrossrefMedlineGoogle Scholar

34.   Andreasen JJ, Mortensen PE, Andersen LI, Arendrup HC, Ilkjaer LB, Kjøller M, Thayssen P.Emergency coronary artery bypass surgery after failed percutaneous transluminal coronary angioplasty.Scand Cardiovasc J. 2000; 34:242–246

36.   U, Levine A, Strang T, Dunning J. If a patient arrests after cardiac surgery is it acceptable to delay cardiopulmonary resuscitation until you have attempted either defibrillation or pacing? Interact Cardiovasc Thorac Surg 2008;7:878-885

37.   Miller AC, Rosati, SF, Suffredini AF, Schrump DS. A Systematic review and pooled analysis of CPR associated cardiovascular and thoracic injuries. Resuscitation 85 (2014 724-731.

38.   Intra-aortic balloon counterpulsation in acute myocardial infarction complicated by cardiogenic shock (IABP-SHOCK II): final 12 month results of a randomised, open-label trial. IABP-SHOCK II Trial Investigators.NEJM;2012,367(14)1287-96, DOI: 10.1056/NEJMoa1208410